# Dry Beetles and Wet Turtles

# Dry Beetles and Wet Turtles

*Charles M. Bump*

ISBN: 1542482518
ISBN 13: 9781542482516

*To all the technologists and other lab personnel I have had the
pleasure of working with over the years.*
*To the infectious-disease specialists and internists, my appreciation and
thanks. There are too many to mention individually, but their work ethic
and dedication have always been an inspiration.*
*To my daughter, Rachel Britton, who has urged me for many years to put
these cases in writing; thanks!*
*And to my wonderful wife, Nancy, who has also told me to just get
busy and do it.*
*My desire is that readers, especially those in the fields of infectious disease and
laboratory medicine, will identify with the cases herein, reflect on those they
could add, and feel the satisfaction that they, too, have contributed to the
health and welfare of their patients.*

# Contents

# Introduction

WHEN IT COMES TO INFECTIOUS diseases, everyone has a story. If it is not about themselves, it is their children, some other member of the family, or a friend. But often it isn't even an infection they are talking about, but some other type of disease. Newspaper reports frequently confuse or mix bacterial infections with viral or parasitic infections. Bacteria are called "bugs" with great regularity even though they are not. Any disease with unknown etiology seems to be a virus, as in "there's a virus going around."

History's take on epidemics is perhaps best told by Hans Zinsser's *Rats, Lice, and History. T*he ongoing pandemic of HIV/AIDS is the best example of a recent historical event, but it is a viral infection, as is the developing H1N1 influenza pandemic. Malaria, a blood-borne, mosquito-transmitted disease, is still an epidemic disease. The increase in tuberculosis around the world is the best example of a bacterial disease affecting current events and eventually history. But these are the big stories and not as meaningful to the individual as the one that has struck at home or perhaps close by. Case histories of unusual diseases make for good stories. Some are contained in modern mystery novels, and others are the basis of short stories. At one time, medical journals would only report large outbreaks of infections, but in more recent times, even "a case of" an organism followed by "and a review of the literature" make the basis of a published report. Whooping cough and measles have made a comeback because of the reluctance of some parents to have their children immunized against them. And that is the result of the allegation that autism is caused by immunizations, although there is no proof of such allegations following extensive investigation.

Unusual circumstances may make for more interesting stories. Berton Roueche published such stories in his classic *Eleven Blue Men*[*] and in many similar books. Paul de Kruif also published several books in this venue, including *Microbe Hunters*. Many of us who have worked in the frontline laboratories of microbiology know of interesting cases of disease or problems in solving the case of an outbreak or cases of rare or unusual organisms causing disease. But these have not caught the attention of academicians or those inclined to turn them into articles suitable for publishing in a scientific journal. During my forty years of work in clinical microbiology laboratories, I have been associated with such cases. Whether arising out of a primitive laboratory in Paraguay or the university-associated infectious-disease department of a major teaching hospital, these are cases you may find interesting and perhaps intellectually stimulating. The stories in this book are all true cases told from my perspective as a clinical microbiologist. They do not contain clinical details from the physician's viewpoint. Actual names of the patients and places are not included to "protect the innocent," and any resemblance to a case you would relate to is purely coincidental. Names are given in some places to give credit to the dedicated, talented, and hardworking technologists and physicians who do deserve the recognition that has eluded them up until now. They have my admiration and respect.

---

[*] Berton Roueche, *Eleven Blue Men* (Boston: Little Brown and Co., 1954).

## CHAPTER 1

# Floors, Mops, and "Tea Kettles"

LATELY, THERE SEEMS TO BE a lot of reinventing the microbiological wheels. There was a scary report on the evening news that (*gasp*) bacteria had been found on the sheets in hospitals and not only on sheets but also on doorknobs, and worst of all, on the mouthpieces of telephones. This was enough to drive those who were even slightly paranoid to the medicine chest to pull out the Lysol, alcohol, or what have you to immediately cleanse such areas. The problem is that this type of information has long been known and is only logical. There is nothing wrong with noting that there are bacteria and viruses on such objects and using disinfectants to clean them. But there is little actual proof that a person can acquire these organisms from such inanimate objects and get an infection from them. A much more likely source of infection is the close proximity of people on public transportation; in the workplace; and in the case of children, in school or at a day-care nursery. Respiratory infections are picked up through the air, not by opening a door or talking on the phone.

For example, one early study showed that the older types of doorknobs made with base metals kill off bacteria, and the bacterial counts on them are much lower than on the new, shiny stainless-steel knobs. Yet we replaced all the old knobs that tarnish, and thus require polishing, with the new ones that are esthetically more pleasing. So why are we now complaining that there are more bacteria on them? Remember, bacteria are everywhere.

In the 1950s, microbiology was a rapidly developing field in hospitals. Infection control was in its infancy. Very few hospitals had an infection-control committee, and fewer made any effort to work on the environmental concerns. Transmission of disease was known, of course, and every effort was made to prevent infections, especially in the operating room (OR). In the sixties, there arose a particular problem that caused a great change in how things were being done, and that was the emergence of serious outbreaks, some fatal, because of the organism *Staphylococcus aureus*: the dreaded "staph." Staph had long been known as a cause of wound infections and such things as boils, but it was appearing in a great number of cases in hospitals, and the later emergence of penicillin-resistant strains resulted in deaths. Epidemiologists were brought in, committees were established, and microbiologists spread out everywhere, taking swabs and doing cultures of virtually anything they could swab. The field of infection control was born, and almost all hospitals organized infection-control committees, run mostly by physicians, laboratory personnel, and a few nurses. Currently, infection-control coordinators are predominantly nurses, but the committees are multidisciplinary. In the 1960s, the committees were busy writing the manuals and developing procedures. Now they are primarily enforcing them and conducting statistical analyses.

## CHAPTER 2

# From Air to Floor to Patients

My first position after finishing a master of science degree in micro-biology was working as an assistant to Dr. Morris Dumoff at McLaren Hospital in Flint, Michigan, where I was assigned special projects, usually in hospital epidemiology. For example, we maintained a stock of staphylo-coccal bacteriophages used in typing *Staphylococcus aureus*, and one of my jobs was to maintain that stock and to type all the staph we isolated. We were particularly looking for strains of phage type 80/81, as this was the strain causing most of the big epidemics across the country. Now, this test-ing is only done at specialized laboratories and only if there has been shown that a threat of a probable outbreak exists.

One of the ways of spreading staph is through the air. Outbreaks in newborn nurseries were particularly devastating, and sometimes a baby ac-quired the organism from the mom during birth and got it all over him- or herself, including in his or her mouth and upper respiratory tract. When these babies cried, they would spray the organism all around and were known as "cloud" babies. One method thought to be useful in removing organisms from the air was ultraviolet light, but this was not particularly useful and was also dangerous. UV light can cause temporary blindness when it is directly shone on one's eyes. (When I was in graduate school, a fellow graduate student and one of his students were temporarily blind-ed by observing an experiment testing the effect of UV light on bacteria. The problem was that the desks in the lab were covered with thick glass, which reflected the UV light back into their eyes. UV light only travels in a straight line and thus does not cover areas shielded from it.)

In our experiment, banks of UV lights were mounted on tall metal poles fastened to a wheeled base. The lights were placed in a corner of a patient room and directed to the center of the room, turned on for fifteen minutes, and turned off. Then they were moved to the next corner, and the process was repeated until all four corners had been covered. Settling plates were placed in the room—up to ten scattered throughout the room—for fifteen minutes before the irradiation was commenced and then again after the completion of the irradiation. The technologist would wear protective covering when entering and leaving the room to minimize the addition of organisms.

There were negligible differences in the "before" and "after" counts. UV lights have seldom been used to disinfect rooms, but recently I have seen advertisements for just this type of setup but did not see studies proving its effectiveness. In my opinion, unless there is corroborating scientific evidence that there is validity in an "improved" UV system, it is a waste of time and money.

## FOGGING

Another method proposed to reduced airborne pathogens was by "fogging" with disinfectants. The fogging apparatus looked like an electric tea-kettle. A disinfectant solution was put into it, and it was placed in a room, plugged in, and turned on, and the door was shut. The fogging apparatus shot a heavy mist of the disinfectant into the air. If this did not eliminate the organisms floating about in the room's atmosphere, then the falling mist would carry them to the floor, or so it was thought. My job was to test it out. I would sample representative sections of the floor before and after fogging by swabbing a controlled area and performing plate counts. We also had an air-sampling device called a slit-sampler and would take air samples. There was no doubt that the fogging reduced the number of organisms in the air, but the number on the floor went up. In other words, the disinfectant was not killing them but simply bringing them to the ground. This meant that once they had dried on the floor, they could probably be recirculated into the air by air currents. We had to find a way to eliminate them on the floor.

One day, as I was taking some "after" samples on the floor, Dr. Dumoff came to see what I was up to and noticed that there was a mop in a bucket nearby that was being used by housekeeping personnel to mop the floors. A disinfectant was always added to the water, so he thought why not mop the floor with the disinfectant and either kill them with the higher concentration used in the mop water or pick them up in the mop water and flush them away. So he mopped it himself, and I took more samples after the mopping was completed. (You don't see many PhDs willing to mop floors.)

We were both shocked with the results. There was little difference between the "before" and "after" fogging counts. The numbers of bacteria on the floor were relatively low and showed a slight increase post fogging. But the results after mopping showed a huge increase in the number of bacteria present, mostly consisting of an organism known as *Pseudomonas aeruginosa*. In other words, the mopping of the floor was inoculating it with large amounts of pseudomonads. This organism can cause disease, most generally urinary-tract infections, but it is also found in wounds, particularly those associated with dirt or water contamination. It is often resistant to many different antibiotics. Rarely does it cause pulmonary disease, but we certainly don't like to see it in large numbers from any clinical source.

Mops were generally used over and over and either hung in the custodian's closet or just left in the mop bucket overnight. During the day, it would not be unusual to see the mop standing in the filled mop bucket. This was a great medium for growth of pseudomonads and similar organisms. The custodial closets were often very warm, and the increased temperature encouraged the growth of pseudomonads. We did not publish these findings, but we did tell other microbiologists we knew of our studies and instituted changes in how mops were handled at McLaren Medical

Center. Similar studies were published, however, and soon regulations were developed regarding mops, such as the maximum number of rooms that could be mopped before the water and mop were changed. Mops could no longer be left overnight and had to be cleaned and disinfected or sterilized. They could not be left in mop water or hung up wet and then reused. I doubt if most people follow such guidelines in their own homes, but it would be good practice.

After several trials, the fogging experiment was deemed not to have been a success, and it was not used further, but the mop experiment led to improved practice. This is not unusual in many fields of science in which one sets out to test an idea only to find it leading to a better one than the one that was intended.

As for the staph problem, although staphylococci are still a major problem, outbreaks like those that occurred in the 1960s are now infrequent. This is probably because of all the changes that have occurred since hospital-infection-control policies have been adopted and the ongoing surveillance that takes place in all hospitals. Presently, the emphasis in on the methicillin-resistant *Staphylococcus aureus*, commonly known as MRSA.

Dedicated infection-control personnel deserve our accolades for the great job they do. This field has also been extended into nursing homes and has helped improve the quality of life there as well.

Airborne organisms can settle out with time, floating down on dust particles to the surface, including the floors. To evaluate the numbers of organisms, we used settling plates, placing agar plates (usually containing sheep blood agar) and removing the lids. We waited a specified length of time, replaced the lids, incubated the plates, and then examined them for growth. The total count of the colonies of bacteria present would be recorded, sometimes including the types of organisms present and the identification of some of them. We would specifically look for the presence of *Staphylococcus aureus*, which is still one of the most frequent causes of nosocomial (hospital-acquired) infection. In the past few years, the problem of resistant bacteria has been a major concern for the medical profession. Specifically, methicillin-resistant *S. aureus* or MRSA are of prominence, owing to their resistance to many of the usual antibiotics prescribed, and are also now found in the general environment besides hospitals.

## MOPPING IN MEXICO

Many years later—in 2007—I went to a hospital in Mexico at their invitation to investigate the cause of an outbreak in a newborn nursery where three infants had become infected with *Pseudomonas* species and one had died. The nursery had recently been rebuilt and was in excellent physical condition. Most of the equipment was new, including the isolettes, and the area was visibly very clean. However, the method used for mopping and cleaning was essentially the same as we had been using years before. There was no standard way of cleaning, although disinfectant was added to the mop water, theoretically in a specified amount. However, the mops were left in the buckets, even overnight, and there was no limit to the area being mopped except in the surgical suites, where each suite was mopped and surfaces cleaned individually. (Here the staff acted in excess at the insistence of one of the surgeons. They cleaned the whole suite—floors and walls included—three times with disinfectants.)

But one of the problems with the disinfectants supplied by the government was that there was no indication of the concentration of the stock disinfectant or how to properly dilute it for use. We sampled several of the mops and mop buckets and found high levels of bacteria including pseudomonads in some and in others essentially sterile conditions. A sampling of the isolette surfaces was also sterile except for a sampling of the air filter, which was loaded with a mixture of organisms resembling that of stool specimens, including *Pseudomonas* species and other gram-negative rods. How this came about could not be determined, but recommendations as to the proper way of mopping were instituted based on standard methods in the United States. One of the recommendations took advantage of the hot temperatures and sunlight in that area of Mexico even in the winter; we had them hang the mops up on lines in the direct sunlight.

The air filters in the isolettes were replaced with new sterile ones and were to be monitored. To my knowledge, no more infants have been infected. The hospital was very cooperative, worked diligently to correct any problems, and should be commended for its actions. Hopefully, the labeling of the concentration of stock disinfectants will be addressed, but the local hospital has no control over that.

## MISCELLANEOUS ENVIRONMENTAL PROBLEMS

Over the years, infection-control staff have had to constantly monitor the cleaning of all areas in the hospital. When an outbreak occurs, the environment is frequently blamed, but in a clear majority of cases, it is personnel, and not the environment, who are the source of the infectious agent. The first thing that needs to be checked out is the causative agent and its normal or usual source. Some organisms are usually found on or in people and are not generally from an environmental source, but others are found in the environment, as with the pseudomonads mentioned above.

As a further example of environmental pseudomonads, we had an increase in urinary-tract infections following cystoscopy and found large numbers of these organisms on the floor and in the floor drain in the surgical suite. Whether they were from the patient or picked up by the patient is some way could not be conclusively determined. *Pseudomonas* species are a common cause of urinary-tract infection. Additional disinfection of the floors and the drain was recommended.

If the organism is part of the commensal flora of humans, then it is prudent to begin to check out who had been in contact with the patient during the incubation period for the infectious agent involved in the case at hand. This can produce a long list of contacts in many cases. But there are ways of reducing the list of personnel needing to be checked for the carrier state of the organism as well as of sampling the personnel. The most common organism is such outbreaks is the notorious *Staphylococcus aureus*, which is a common resident of human skin and nose. Swabs of the nares and hands can lead to finding staph. Staphylococci can then be typed to determine if the isolate is the same type as the one causing the infection.

## CHAPTER 3

# Sporotrichosis in Owosso, Michigan

SPOROTRICHOSIS IS A DISEASE CAUSED by the dimorphic fungus *Sporothrix schenckii*. It is perhaps one of the most beautiful organisms when viewed in its filamentous form under a microscope, as it has delicate filaments with clusters of flower-like spores. It has often been called rose-grower's disease and is associated with scratches from rose bushes. However, this may be misleading; it can be acquired from any type of scratch, as the organism can be found in peat moss and soil.

One day, a patient came into the Owosso Memorial Hospital with a request from Dr. Terpstra that we culture a lesion on the back of the patient's hand that resembled a boil. The probability was that this was a staphylococcal infection. However, I noted that the lesion was open and shallow, and I could feel hard lymph nodes along the patient's arm. This is suspicious for sporotrichosis. A Gram stain did not reveal the typical clusters of staphylococci, but some small, cigar-shaped structures were observed: this is indicative of "sporo," so a culture was also set up for fungi. Now staph grow quickly. In eighteen to twenty-four hours, you can expect to see them growing on a culture plate, but sporo can take three to five days to appear. It has a white, leathery appearance which gradually turns black. The culture plates for bacteria did not show any growth as expected, but growth as described above did, in fact, happen. Microscopic examination of the growth proved it to be probable *Sporothrix schenckii*. The recommended treatment for sporotrichosis at that time was supersaturated potassium iodide (SSKI), which was added to milk, as it has a bitter taste. And it had to be given for a long period before a cure was achieved. Once we had identified this organism, we contacted Dr. Terpstra, who started the patient on SSKI. Because of the rarity of this disease, we inquired into the history of the patient, hoping to determine where he might have picked up the organism. The patient worked for a company in Ovid, Michigan, that packaged rose bushes. The company would receive train-car loads of bare-root rose bushes from out west (Arizona and New Mexico), wrap the roots in sphagnum moss, and then wrap them in wax paper for a chain of stores with garden shops. The patient had doubtless been scratched many times, and of course, these were rose bushes, so rose-grower's disease was the logical conclusion.

We contacted the company and arranged to go there and get cultures of the peat moss and anything else that might contain the infectious agent. The bushes were kept in the dark to prevent early sprouting before they were ready for sale. There was plenty of moss to culture. We also noted that, at the sink for washing up, there were bottles of betadine, a form of iodine that is used for disinfection. Although not proven to my knowledge, I believe iodine may help prevent more cases of sporotrichosis. The wonder was not having a case of sporotrichosis from this site but that there were not more of them.

The cultures we obtained did grow out organisms similar to *Sporotrichum schenckii* but not identical. This organism is one of those dimorphic fungi that grow as a yeast form at thirty-seven degrees Celsius or in infected animals and as a filamentous fungus at room temperature. The isolates we obtained would not convert to the yeast phase from the filamentous form, which we found on several plates inoculated with the sphagnum moss.

I come from a family of florists, and my mother's hands were crisscrossed with scars caused by rose thorns, but she never got sporotrichosis. Cut roses are not contaminated with peat or sphagnum moss. I know many people who work around, and with roses, who have never gotten this disease. The real concern is with the moss, although it seems that whenever a case of sporo is found, a search is made for the rose connection.

I had another case when I was working in Massachusetts, an itinerant farmhand who had extensive sporo. He was following the crops from south to north, living in temporary quarters as he traveled. Most of his work involved digging for potatoes, where he would encounter the soil. After his diagnosis, his case history was obtained with careful questioning about a rose connection. And sure enough, he did recall that, while in Delaware, he'd had to climb to the top of his trailer home to fix the TV antenna and had put the ladder over some climbing rose bushes to get there. So, you see, there was the rose connection! Having found this, the clinicians were happy to make the diagnosis: rose-grower's disease.

The second case in Owosso involved a former city councilman who appeared in Dr. Park's office with a lesion on his hand. Dr. Park sent him to us with a request for a culture of the lesion. This patient also had the hard lymph nodes up his arm and a history of having scratched his hand while trimming and cleaning out the hedges at his house. We set up the cultures, including those for fungi, and several days later grew out sporo. The patient was started on SSKI, and we thought that would take care of this case. We were wrong. It seemed the naysayer friends of the patient thought we, being in a community hospital in a rural area, did not know what we were doing and suggested that he go to a nearby major university-associated medical center for further evaluation. Since the lesion was on the knuckle of a finger, the patient was referred to the orthopedic clinic and not to the infectious-disease clinic. The physicians there thought it was a staph infection, stopped the SSKI, started him on antistaphylococcal therapy, and sent him home.

I received a call from Dr. Park later. He asked me if I was sure of the identification and related to me the story the patient had told him regarding his university experience. Later, the patient, whom I know, also called me and told me how I must have been mistaken. I asked him if he was getting better on the therapy he was on. Well, not really, was the answer. I assured him I had the organism on a culture plate in my laboratory, and he ought to go back to the SSKI. (I also called the university and found out that they had not obtained a culture and had not really evaluated him for sporo. I offered to send them the culture I had, but they chose not to receive it.) Several weeks later, the patient stopped by to show me how nicely his hand was healing with the SSKI therapy. He also said he was spreading the word to his friends and acquaintances that we knew what we were doing.

It was not long after that, when another patient showed up at my door with a story much like the second patient's. In fact, they were friends, and they had compared cases before he came to the doctor for treatment of his hand lesion. He had been working at his cottage up north, also cleaning out bushes. Buoyed by his friend's successful treatment after the sporo diagnosis and his renewed faith in our local medical community, our third case was soon cured.

This is a prime example of times that the adage "when you hear hoofbeats, think horses not zebras" does not apply. It is generally true that the most common condition (in this case, staphylococcal infections) should be expected, but who knows when a circus may come to town, and a zebra could have escaped. The rarity of sporotrichosis does not mean one should not check for the telltale string of hard lymph nodes proceeding up the arm.

Note: Since these cases, the SSKI has been replaced with specific antifungal agents, which are more powerful and specific but also more expensive than the saturated iodine.

CHAPTER 4

# Ectoparasites

ECTOPARASITES ARE THE LARGER MULTICELLULAR organisms that get on people and infest them. They, unlike bacteria, may include true bugs, most commonly on the head, body, and pubis. (Pubic lice are called crabs.) Head lice cause more stress and discomfort than many other, more dangerous organisms, whether they are found in a school, hospital, or clinic setting. Head lice in a school population creates instant action from treatment to notification of parents and mass checking to find and identify other infested students. Some schools will even close for a day or two to "disinfect" the entire school before allowing students back in. My father once told me head lice were very common in his youth, and no one was surprised or alarmed when a child was found with them. And the treatment was quite simple: shampoo with kerosene! I understand this really is effective, inexpensive although odoriferous, and easy to do. Of course, it is probably not used except in remote areas, as there are several other agents used. These are more expensive, some requiring a physician's prescription, but more sophisticated. During treatment, it is still essential to carefully groom the patient with a fine comb to find and remove the nits, which are the eggs of the louse. (I'm certain many readers will recall pictures of the careful grooming practiced by great apes.)

Body lice are very common in colder climates, particularly during wartimes or during other calamities resulting in crowds of homeless people and refugees. This is probably because of the fact that refugees often wear multiple layers of clothing and are unable to change them or bathe for long periods of time. During World War II, arriving emigrants were dusted down with large amounts of DDT powder to kill the lice. The disease typhus is a louse-borne disease. There are several other rickettsial diseases that are transmitted by lice and fleas.

Pubic lice or crabs are most commonly found in the genital region of the body but may also be found in eyelashes. (I won't go into that!) The shape of these parasites is quite distinctive, easily recognized and differentiated from the body/head louse by the trained observer. Sexual transmission is the most common means of spreading the infestation. Pubic lice do not fly or jump from person to person, and close intimate contact is required, although it is possible to pick them up by getting into a bed very soon after it has been used by an infested person.

This leads me to another case. One day I received a call from a man who identified himself as our hospital's attorney requesting some information about pubic lice, including the life cycle, which I supplied. He then told me that the hospital was being sued by a former patient who had become infested with pubic lice while in our hospital. She declared it must have come from the sheets not being changed between patients. She demanded five thousand dollars, which the hospital had refused to pay. I would be an expert witness on behalf of the hospital, as it was going to a jury trial. Before the trial, I met with the attorney over lunch, and he instructed me as to how the trial would go and what questions he would be putting to me on the witness stand. It was a straightforward case. We had a witness who would testify she had entered the patient's room to find a man—the woman's significant other—climbing out of the bed.

I went to the courthouse at the appointed time and waited outside the courtroom, as witnesses are not permitted to hear prior testimony. I waited all morning, a very long time for what should have been a short case. After lunch, I was brought in and put on the witness stand, sworn in, and then informed I was considered a hostile witness, so the plaintiff's attorney would be allowed to question me first. I looked at our attorney, and he just shrugged his shoulders. The questions were concise: basically asking about the life cycle of lice, whether they could fly, and how they would get from person to person. After I had answered his questions—our attorney had none—I was sent back to the hall, as it was determined I might be recalled.

The jury had seven members. Later, I learned that a member of the jury had confessed to having been infested with crabs previously. Our attorney thought he'd be a good person to have on the jury.

All afternoon I waited, watching the activities and reading to while away the time. A lot of money was being spent on this case, probably more than the five thousand dollars sought in settlement, but there was a principle to uphold. Around 5:00 p.m., the door to the courtroom burst open, and the crowd surged out. Finally, our attorney came out and over to where I stood. He was laughing, so I knew it had to be good.

"What happened?" was my question.

"The judge dismissed the case and chewed out the plaintiff for a frivolous case."

It turned out that the plaintiff's boyfriend had been put on the stand and confessed to having crabs and having been in bed with her at the hospital. And of course, that was the close personal contact I described as being the most common means of contracting crabs. The plaintiff, instead of being embarrassed, thought she was still entitled and declared she'd never come to our hospital again.

Our attorney apologized to me for not being able to inform me beforehand that I would be declared a hostile witness but said I had done well. I hope he had informed our CEO, although I never heard from him regarding the case. My immediate supervisor was quite happy with the way it had turned out, and my day away from the lab was well spent. At least I got a free lunch at one of the prime restaurants in town (no doubt billed to the hospital).

One day when I was sitting in my office and half the lab was on lunch break, one of my techs slipped in, shut the door, and sat in the chair in front of my desk. He held out a small screw-capped test tube.

"Are these what I think they are?"

I took the tube. In it were several small, reddish-brown crawling insects. Before stating what I thought, I took out a magnifying glass. I could make out the squat body with the enlarged front pair of legs characteristic of crabs. "If you think they are crabs, I would agree with you. Where did you get them?"

He looked out the window of the door then turned and said "Off of me."

"Guess you better get some lotion and get rid of them. Sorry."

"But that's only part of the problem."

"Why's that?"

"It's where or who I got them from."

"Well, I guess that is a personal problem, and I can't help you there."

"It will be part of your problem maybe. You see I got them from…" And he named one of the young ladies working with him in the lab.

"That is a problem, but if you are certain…"

"Oh, I am. I haven't had another sex partner in a long time, and I got these just after spending a weekend with her."

"You need to tell her and make certain she is treated too."

"You think we could be a problem to anyone else in the lab?"

"Not unless you get as personal with them as you did with her."

He sighed, took his crabs, and left. A few days later, he reported back to me that he'd had a stormy session with her as she tried to tell him he must have given them to her. But he had found out from her good friend that she was somewhat promiscuous and had frequent partners some of whom had unsavory backgrounds. It took a while, but the tense atmosphere in the lab, which had been felt by all, finally abated, and he reported all the crabs had been eliminated.

This was the second case of crabs I knew about that occurred between coworkers—not, however, in the same hospital—and both were resolved satisfactorily.

Ticks are another common ectoparasitic animals, with humans being incidental. They also may transmit rickettsial diseases, such as Rocky

Mountain spotted fever. The most common tick is the dog tick, although the lone star tick is also common in some parts of the country. More recently, a spirochetal organism (*Borrelia*), which is transmitted by the deer tick, was found to cause a skin disease with systemic symptoms. It is called Lyme disease, after the name of the town in Connecticut where it was first described. Deer ticks are much smaller than dog ticks and are easily identified by a trained technologist. The appearance of Lyme disease in Wisconsin and Minnesota was perplexing at first, but it has been shown that the deer tick catches rides on migrating wading birds, some of which may well have traveled from New England to the Midwest. Although often suspected, very few confirmed cases of Lyme disease are found in Michigan, as there are fewer deer ticks there.

During the time I worked in Massachusetts, we had a case of Rocky Mountain spotted fever identified both clinically and serologically. But it was unusual in that the young boy who had it was living in Florida at the time and had been there longer than the incubation time for the tick-borne disease. Now Rocky Mountain spotted fever (RMSF) was first identified in the Rockies and received its name as a result, but now more cases of RMSF are found in other areas of the country, including the Cape Cod region of Massachusetts where this patient's home was located, but not in Florida. Either there had been an extraordinarily long incubation time, which would be a new finding, or there was some other reason.

It did not take too long for the epidemiologist to find out the reason. It seems the little boy had gotten homesick for his dog, who had remained home when they left for Florida. The grandfather had plenty of money and a great heart for his grandson and had flown the dog to Florida. The dog had been infested with ticks and slept in the same bed with the boy. An examination of the boy had revealed ticks that had been removed, but by that time, he had been infested. End of story.

But maybe not. We had a rare case of tick paralysis, although I was not personally involved. A young boy had become paralyzed and no cause had been found. Ours was at least the third hospital the child had been admitted to, and he was close to death. One of the physicians with a suspicion in mind conducted a thorough examination of the boy and found in the nape of his neck, completely hidden in his hair, a greatly enlarged tick. He carefully removed it, sent it to the lab for identification, and waited. Very quickly, the boy began to recover. Ticks elaborate a toxin, which was causing the paralysis. A very good reason to be careful in examining children when you live or vacation in an area where there are plenty of ticks.

## FLIES IN THE HOSPITAL

More unusual are diseases caused by flies, including the common housefly. In fact, fly larvae (maggots) are used to debride dead tissue from gangrenous wounds. We observed one case of maggots in a newborn child whose mother had not removed the bellyband. When she showed up in the doctor's office with the infested baby, the doctor unwound the baby's bellyband which, by the way, exuded a strong odor, and found a large number of maggots in the umbilicus. The maggots were sent to our laboratory for identification. Each species of fly can be identified in the larval stage by examining the rear end of the larva for distinctive markings or by allowing the larva to develop to the adult stage, which is simpler to identify, at least by the amateur. Sometimes you must feed the larva and wait while it goes through the stages to become the adult fly. We did this once by putting hamburger in a petri dish along with the maggots and waiting until the adult fly emerged. In the case above, we identified the larvae as those of the green bottle fly.

No one likes to see flies in his or her home, so you can imagine the stress caused by the appearance of flies in an operating room, especially during surgery. Once that occurs, there is an immediate search for and elimination of the source and any flies present. However, this is not always easy. It becomes easier if you know the species of fly involved and its natural history.

A surgical nurse arrived in our laboratory one day carrying a container with several flies captured in a surgical suite and asked for our help in determining the source. We examined the surgical wing carefully, but we could not find the source, and although the flies were being killed as fast as they came, they continued to appear. We decided to take some of the flies to Michigan State University department of entomology for identification. To our relief, the flies were rapidly identified and their characteristics made known. We learned these flies laid their eggs in soil, and when they hatched out into the adult stage, they would climb the nearest object, tree, or building to the highest point and then fly away. The increased height gave them a head start and a longer range of flight. In climbing up a building, they would sometimes find their way through holes in the screens of the windows or gaps under them. In our institution, the operating floor was in the top floor of the building, and the flies had found ways to get into the rooms. The application of appropriate lethal agents to the soil at the base of the building under the windows of the surgical suites was effective, and the flies were eliminated. The windows were also resealed to eliminate points of entrance.

Several years later, the same problem arose in another hospital but with a different species of fly. These were triangle- or delta-shaped flies with transparent black wings and were identified as sewer flies. After an extensive search, we were unable to find the source, and it was increasingly perplexing and frustrating to everyone involved. The number of flies getting into the operating rooms was increasing, and surgeons threatened to close them down until the flies could be eliminated. This, of course, would cause considerable financial loss to the hospital, as well as delay in treatment for the patients.

One day, the infection-control coordinator and the maintenance supervisor were walking down a basement corridor, and the ICC happened to notice a small square door high on the wall of the hallway. This door, she was told, opened to an area under the kitchen where the drains to the sinks were located. She insisted it be opened; the drains led to sewers, and these were sewer flies. A ladder was brought, and the door was opened and immediately slammed shut. The interior swarmed with thousands and thousands of flies. A "bug bomb" was obtained, inserted, and exploded. After the appropriate amount of time had passed, the results were observed. When the door was reopened, it was discovered that one or more of the drains had been leaking and spilling the dirty water—sewage of a sort—into the tunnel. Flies had been living and dying there for some time, resulting in an accumulation of dead flies several feet thick. They had to be shoveled out and removed, the tunnel cleaned, and the drains repaired to eliminate the problem. Again, the identification of the flies was instrumental in the correction of the problem. The OR was safe again.

Over the years, it was rare but not unusual to receive roundworms in the laboratory. These were almost always the classic intestinal roundworm, which sometimes results in obstruction of the intestinal tract or in appendicitis. In one case, a shiny, new unlabeled gallon paint can was brought to our lab. In it were thirteen long *Ascaris* worms the parents had retrieved from their child's stool specimens. In another case, I did identify an earthworm a small child had apparently eaten unknown to his parents, who were understandably alarmed about finding the worm in the stool specimen. At least they were relieved it was not a roundworm requiring treatment of the child.

Sometimes ectoparasites are false. Once I received a plastic bag filled with small pieces of clear scotch tape folded over on themselves. The patient, believing she was crawling with small bugs, had used the tape to "catch" and remove them. She had requested the physician to identify them, but when we examined them carefully under the microscope, no parasites were to be found. So confident was the patient that she did have bugs crawling on her, she submitted another twenty or thirty pieces of tape, which were again examined to no avail. We suspect her next appointment was with her psychiatrist.

I had a personal case of an ectoparasite while serving as a student summer missionary in Paraguay. I had been chosen to go to Paraguay and work in the Hospital Bautista in Asuncion for three months. During that time, I worked on developing the microbiology laboratory as well as doing other assigned tasks, visiting mission sites, and having the opportunity of enjoying the beautiful country. But after being there for a month or so, I began to experience a pain in my second toe and saw a black spot just under the nail that was surrounded by angry red skin. I went to see our pediatrician in his office, as he was the only American doctor there at the time, and showed him my foot. He gave a little laugh and said I had a picca—a type of fly that would lay eggs under the toenail. The eggs had hatched with the resultant larvae burrowing there and growing at my expense. With a little local anesthetic and judicious use of a scalpel blade, the maggot was soon removed. One more souvenir of my visit.

## CHAPTER 5

# Legionnaires' Disease

Now THERE IS NOTHING LIKE a large nationwide epidemic, no matter what causes it, to get people excited. And if there are epidemics and the causative agent cannot be found, that makes it even more exciting. In the 1960s and 1970s, there were several small epidemics of respiratory infections at different locations around the country for which no cause was found. An early one occurred in Pontiac, Michigan, and became known as Pontiac fever, and other epidemics throughout the country created a stir in the medical world. Serum from patients and, in some cases, tissues or other specimens were collected and stored in deep freezers in the hope that someday they could be used to determine if the epidemics were related. And if a new causative agent tissue could be recultured or analyzed by other means, we could determine if the specimen contained that agent. Then, following a convention of the American Legion in Philadelphia, there was another such epidemic among the people who had attended the convention, which was named Legionnaires' disease. But no definitive agent was found. Many laboratories, including the Centers for Disease Control in Chamblee, Georgia, had tried unsuccessfully to isolate an organism using all types of culture media, tissue cultures, and animals. Eventually an organism was isolated in tissue cultures.

During the months following the original outbreak, a patient developed a similar clinical picture and was admitted to McLaren General Hospital in Flint, Michigan. A specimen of pleural fluid was sent to the microbiology laboratory along with sputum specimens, and at first, as with other cases, no organism was found except for the usual respiratory flora in the sputum culture. After several days, the technologist, Dorothy Broomfield, working on the culture of the pleural fluid noticed very small, almost transparent, colonies on the chocolate agar plate. (Chocolate agar is not made with chocolate but is named for the chocolate color that results from the change in blood used to make the plate owing to the high temperature in its preparation. It's analogous to your steak turning brown when it is cooked). The results of the Gram stain she prepared of the culture revealed very faintly stained gram-negative rods, but they could not be identified further by the usual means for this type of organism. A subculture was sent to the Michigan Department of Public Health in Lansing, Michigan. Technologists there could not identify it either, and the culture was forwarded on to the CDC.

At the time, the CDC was working with an organism that had been isolated in tissue cultures from patients diagnosed with Legionnaires' disease. It was also a tiny, faintly stained gram-negative rod and was considered to be the probable agent of Legionnaires' disease. The McLaren patient's clinical signs and symptoms were consistent with this syndrome; therefore, the two organisms were compared and determined to be the same. But what interested the microbiologists at the CDC more was the fact that the sample from McLaren had been isolated on routine culture media, but they were unable to grow it on the chocolate agar plates they used. They began a study comparing the media McLaren was using to the medium the CDC used. Extract of yeast was included in the McLaren chocolate agar but not in the CDC's, and this had an essential nutrient required for the growth of the isolate. Further investigation showed a requirement for cysteine. Subsequently, another medium was developed that did not use blood but had activated charcoal, cysteine, and other ingredients that promoted the growth of the organism in almost a pure state and with a rather distinctive bluish color, making isolation of the organism much easier. This organism was eventually named *Legionella pneumophila* in recognition of the epidemic in members of the American Legion and to indicate its predilection for (love of) the lungs.

An epidemiologic investigation at the site in Philadelphia and in similar outbreaks throughout the country concluded that this organism is present in fresh water in many parts of the world and actually resides within algal cells. How it got to people from the water source was the next mystery to resolve. There were also several closely related species found and identified, some of which can also cause human disease, but the most commonly found isolate in infected patients was *Legionella pneumophila*. The microbiologist at McLaren Hospital became involved with characterizing the organism and was an author of one of the early papers regarding clinically isolating it. He became ill and was hospitalized; during his hospital stay, he also developed characteristics of legionellosis, and this probably contributed to his death. Because of his early involvement and to honor his long career in the field of clinical microbiology, a subsequent species of *Legionella* was named after him: *Legionella dumoffii*.

He was not the only patient to acquire this infection while in the hospital (this is known as a hospital-acquired or nosocomial infection), and an intense investigation was conducted to find the source. Because the organism was waterborne, the water was tested throughout the hospital in faucets, drains, showerheads, and fountains, and it was found in multiple sites. Once it has colonized water pipes, it is most difficult to eradicate. The organism is resistant to the normal levels of chorine that are routinely added to drinking water.

Patients were likely acquiring the Legionnaires' bacillus by inhaling the organism while taking a shower or perhaps by aspirating it while drinking the water. This organism is not very virulent (i.e., capable of producing disease), but patients whose immune systems are being challenged by other causes have an increased chance of picking up an infection. It was obviously necessary to eliminate the organism from the water and pipes throughout the medical center. The decision was made to try superheating the water.

One floor was chosen for a test, as the water supplying it could be heated separately from that on the other floors. It would be necessary to keep patients from using the showers and faucets during the time the water was heated to prevent accidental scalding. On the day of the trial, maintenance and other personnel were assigned to watch the bathrooms and to turn on the showers and hot water faucets to allow the water to run and, they hoped, disinfect the terminal ends of the water lines as well as the pipes themselves. Pipes get coated with organic and inorganic chemical compounds that also decrease the flow of water, providing a place to harbor bacteria. However, one little detail had been overlooked. The temperature the water was raised to generated huge clouds of steam. All hospitals are equipped with smoke detectors, and before anyone realized, the fire alarms on that floor began going off. The alarm system is also connected to the nearest fire station, and within minutes, the fire engines began pulling up to the hospital, much to the embarrassment of all concerned. Although this did prove to eradicate the organism in the pipes tested, the hospital decided not to continue using it because of all the difficulties and time required. Also, the organism was found in the incoming water, so just superheating the water would not stop its future colonization of the pipes. But higher levels of chlorine could be added to the incoming water.

Controlled amounts of chlorine would be added through attachments in the water mains to increase the total parts per million (ppm) to a level known to kill the *Legionella* organism. The chlorine level would be monitored daily at first and then, if successful, would be monitored weekly and perhaps only monthly. It was a reasonable plan, but complications soon arose. McLaren had grown over the years of its existence, and with the additions to the building, there were found to be two water mains entering the hospital. Chlorine would have to be added to both of them. This program began, and both the level of chlorine and the presence of the organism were monitored. This experiment was successful. The high levels of chlorine did eradicate the organism in the water, but with a loud cry of complaint from many people in the facility about the strong odor of chlorine. It smelled like you were near a swimming pool, and many noted the taste of chlorine in the drinking water.

Now chlorine added to water results in an increase in acidity. Hydrochloric acid (HCl) is a strong acid, too. This acid began to act on the seams of the copper water pipes, and multiple leaks began to appear throughout the hospital. Therefore, the level of chlorine had to be reduced. However, the length of time the high levels of chlorine had been used was sufficient to eliminate the organism from the water. The hospital concluded that a slightly elevated level of chlorine would be sufficient to remove the organism and established a program to monitor the chlorine level and to culture samples of water for *Legionella pneumophila* from several sites throughout the hospital monthly where it had been found earlier.

The program worked well. For months, the cultures were consistently negative. But one day, the technologist processing those cultures came to me, plate in hand, and reported positive cultures for the agent. What had happened?

The first thing to check was the level of chlorine in the water. It was gone. No chlorine was detected. The hospital initiated an investigation. We learned that the chlorine in the city's drinking water was added in one plant on the east side of the city, and we were, at that time, virtually on the far end of the water lines. The farther you are from the source of the chlorine, the greater the chance the levels will be lower, since the chlorine would dissipate along the way or chemically react with the solids coating the water pipes. But it should not be reduced to zero. Our infection-control coordinator made a personal call to the water treatment plant and talked to the personnel there. He learned that the person who was responsible for the addition and monitoring of the chlorine had gone on a three-week vacation, and the person covering that job didn't know or didn't add the chlorine. The official contact with the water department resulted in a denial of this. But the water department did not know that we monitored the level of chlorine at the hospital, and no one could come up with a plausible reason that our testing would show a zero level. This was an impasse that was never, to my knowledge, resolved.

Neither party was happy with the situation. The hospital continued to monitor the chlorine level (and I believe it still goes on), and up until the time I left, there was not another time that the chlorine level was not maintained. The water supplying the city at that time came from Detroit, which got it from the Detroit River. *Legionella pneumophila* is found in water throughout the Great Lakes along with other related species, although in low numbers, so there is a very low risk of infecting people. But when the water is found in places where the organism can grow to high concentrations along with its commensal agent—algae—then it can become a danger to people, especially those with reduced immune status. Aerosolizing of water so the particles are very small and can reach the ends of the lungs greatly increases the chance of someone becoming infected.

But this was not the end of the story. Even several years later, we still had patients developing pulmonary disease owing to *Legionella pneumophila*, and we could not find the source. The water was clear of the infectious agent. We did determine that almost all the cases were coming from one floor in the older original wing of the hospital. I continued to make rounds of the patient areas of the hospital, looking for possible sites and checking out the floors and rooms where the infected patients had been. One day, I was walking down the stairwell and looked out the window, which was higher than the roof of the contiguous central portion of the hospital. I noticed a cloud of steam blowing across the roof, but this was January. Where did the steam originate? The heating source for the hospital was some distance away. Then I noticed that the steam was blowing off an air-conditioning tower, but why would an air-conditioning unit be running in the cold of winter? I located the maintenance director, and he told me that unit served operating rooms on the floor below. The OR lights generated enough heat to require cooling to keep the rooms at a comfortable level.

We went up to the roof to collect samples of the water and the slime coating the wood slats of the cooling tower. A stiff breeze was blowing from the east—unusual for that time of year—and the steam was blowing toward the west and directly into the air intake for the part of the hospital supplying the floor where the *Legionella* patients were found. The cultures were loaded with the causative agent. We had finally found our source. The tower was closed, other means were found to cool the ORs, and eventually, the whole air-conditioning unit was removed and our problem eliminated. No more cases were found. We had solved our mystery.

This is another example of how a little detective work is used to solve medical problems. To me, for one, epidemiology is one of the most interesting and exciting areas of medicine.

Finally, using serologic methods, many of the small epidemics like Pontiac fever (which was not too far from Flint) were studied and compared with legionellosis and found to be the same or closely related. Legionellosis is now quite rare; the use of chlorine in water, the monitoring of levels, and the elimination or controlled use of cooling towers and other stagnant water sources have removed the source of this organism.

CHAPTER 6

# Dried Beetles and Wet Turtles

WORKING IN LARGE MEDICAL CENTERS with major university connections has wide implications in the practice of clinical microbiology. For one, there are usually specialized clinics handling rare and unusual conditions. Patients who have a disease that has not been diagnosed at smaller institutions will be referred to these clinics and the experts associated with them. It is quite likely that the infectious-disease clinic will see patients with unusual, rare, or even unknown conditions. But at times some very unusual conditions can arise at other clinics where the patient is not suspected of having an infectious disease. I worked for several large university-based institutions and, thus, did see a number of such cases.

One of these came from the "failure-to-thrive" clinic. This clinic received babies who, after birth, did not develop at the expected rate for a variety of reasons. It is the task of the clinicians handling these patients to find out the reason and correct it. They had a list of suspected conditions or reasons for these failure-to-thrive babies, as most specialized clinics do. One of these was that the baby might be unable to process the food he or she was given, including the mother's milk. If the food traveled too rapidly through the baby's system, the baby could fail to digest or assimilate the food.

Several methods had been developed to determine the length of time it took for food to go through the baby. One of the methods was to have the baby ingest a capsule that contained a thread tied in some manner outside the baby's mouth and held there until the capsule was delivered from the terminal end. The thread could be pulled back at any time, especially if the capsule became stuck somewhere in the alimentary tract. The thread could be examined microscopically if necessary to see what might have attached to it. It could also be cultured for organisms, but this was rarely done.

Normally, this clinic did not see any pathogenic organisms as the cause of failure to thrive, but then an unusual event happened. Many of the babies developed severe diarrhea. This should not have been happening and required immediate action to determine the cause. Stool (what feces is called in microbiology laboratories) cultures were obtained from all the affected babies. In quick order (two to three days), the causative agent for the diarrhea was found to be a biotype of *Salmonella* species named *S. cubana*.

There are more than twenty-two hundred bioserotypes of *Salmonella*, although not more than three or four distinct species. By typing the isolates, you can determine if they are the same from patient to patient; if they are, it would be certain that the organisms came from the same source. In this outbreak, we cultured the same biotype from every baby with diarrhea, but the next question was: what was the source? The isolates were isolated and identified in the main laboratory, but I was directed to determine the source.

I first reviewed the case histories to see if any of the babies had arrived at the clinic with diarrhea that could have been transmitted to the other babies by personnel. None fit that criterion.

Could any of the staff have been the source? The easy part was questioning the staff, including incidental personnel such as the dietary workers and janitorial, nursing, and medical staffs. Not one had recently experienced diarrhea. Now there is such a thing as a carrier state, in which a person has an organism in his or her body but does not show clinical conditions. To determine this, everyone would have had to submit a stool specimen for culture. With *Salmonella*, the most likely source would require close attention and no incidental contact. As we prepared to do this, we determined that the serotype *S. cubana* was quite rare, and only a few isolates were found in the state we were in. It seemed unlikely that personnel were involved. A quick check of travel histories indicated that no one had traveled recently, and no outbreak of the isolate had been reported.

Now our task was to determine where the organism was hiding and its original source. Since *Salmonella* are most likely to have come from food and water, it was necessary to sample and culture all food and water sources that had been used for the babies. This included the milk, the formula, and the water used to reconstitute the formula. This also included mother's milk samples. (Human breast milk is donated and maintained under proper conditions for babies whose mothers cannot provide it.)

None of the sources tested positive for *Salmonella* or any other pathogen. We had to go back and review our epidemiology studies to see if we could find another possible source. A careful review showed that all the babies who had diarrhea had been tested to determine how long food took to go through their bodies using a capsule filled with a bright red dye called carmine red. This dye was widely used for a variety of procedures in which an easily visible marker was needed. Such dyes are also used in foods such as Jell-O. The capsule dissolved quickly, releasing dye into the intestinal track, and the stools were examined for the appearance of the red color. A rapid appearance would indicate insufficient time for absorbance of nutrients. We obtained several of the dye capsules and cultured them by several methods for the presence of organisms, including *Salmonella*. The outsides of the capsules were cultured separately from the dye and were negative, but a pure culture of the *Salmonella cubana* recovered from the babies was obtained from the dye itself. We had solved the problem of the diarrhea but still needed to find out how the *Salmonella* got into the dye.

We contacted the company that made the dye capsules and learned that dye was made by grinding up dried beetles, which are found generally in two places in the world: Peru and the Canary Islands. People would collect the cochineal beetles off plants, allow them to die, dry them, separate the extraneous material associated with them, and sell them to makers of dye. To confirm and hopefully find the original source, we decided to go to the Canary Islands and Peru to finish the study. Although I had hoped to go, it ended up that the director of our laboratory and the clinician in charge of the clinic were sent, all expenses paid, to the Canary Islands. Another team was sent to Peru. They explained the problem and conducted careful studies. Some of the beetles in Peru had been infected with the organism, although no other source was determined. There were many steps in the dye-making process during which the product could have become contaminated. Cultures of the machinery in Peru grew out heavy growth of the *Salmonella*, although the original source was not located. This problem and its solution were eventually published. Proper safeguards were put in place and additional quality control measures instituted to prevent this from occurring again.

Once the contaminated dye capsules were eliminated and certified *Salmonella*-free capsules put into use, the incidence of diarrhea was also eliminated. Carmine red dye was added to the list of possible sources for *Salmonella* infections.

This was only one incidence in which *Salmonella* caused an outbreak of diarrhea in our hospital. Our technologists were frequently the first to notice an increase or potential cluster of cases, which may indicate an outbreak. At the time of this outbreak, the field of hospital-based epidemiology was in its infancy. Infection-control committees were not found in many hospitals, and the position of infection-control coordinator (several different titles have been used) was a new and developing one. Our hospital was a leader in this field, and we had a full-time infection-control coordinator but no support staff. This man had been brought in from another state, as he had some training and background in epidemiology, and reported to the director of our laboratory, who was a PhD microbiologist. On a daily basis, he would come through the lab and pick up any information that needed to be evaluated for potential outbreaks and then investigate them.

An increase in any isolated pathogen needed careful study but especially *Staphylococcus aureus.* We did not expect to find an outbreak of *Salmonella* in the hospital, but all isolates of pathogenic organisms were reported to the state departments of public health, which would then be on the lookout for epidemics.

Any case of salmonellosis in the pediatric department of a hospital is a serious problem. The source of such infections must be determined before they can be eliminated. Rates of nosocomial infections for any hospital should be available to the public, but this will be the subject of another chapter.

After identifying a problem—an outbreak of diarrhea—the pediatric department personnel were put on notice, and immediate action was taken to isolate those patients to prevent the spread of the infection. Patients were cohorted. No new patients were admitted to rooms with infected patients until the patients were discharged and the rooms completely and thoroughly disinfected. Stool precautions were established, and contaminated materials, especially those in contact with stool, were carefully removed and disinfected.

Epidemiologic studies, including medical histories of all staff, were done as with the cases presented above. Again, no source was found. Then began a complete examination of the physical attributes of the rooms and environment the sick children were in. Of course, we had to consider all water, food, and any other materials the patients were consuming or would be in contact with. This was done, but no infectious agents were found, and yet new cases continued to develop.

Because this was a pediatric unit, there were many things not generally found in patient wards: toys of all sorts, flowers, and cages of animals. These were all examined, and there was no source until someone found a small aquarium that held several small painted turtles. Children were permitted to pick these up and handle them if they desired. Several specimens of the water were sent down, and I was given the task of doing the epidemiology cultures for enteric pathogens, specifically *Salmonella.*

When testing water, since there might be only a very few organisms in it, we must test a large sample. At that time, we would use a pipette to pick up the sample and transfer it to culture media. This is not a problem with tap water or other such water sources, as there are no large particles in them. This wasn't true with the "turtle water," which contained quite a bit of material that would plug the end of the pipette. After trying several different ways to sample the water, I found that by reversing the ends of the pipette and sucking up the water through the mouth end, I could get a sufficient sample. Almost all, if not all, the turtle-water samples grew *Salmonella* species that were of the same serotype as those obtained from the infected patients. But this did not definitively identify the source. Was it the water, the turtles, or someone's contaminated hands?

The water used in the aquarium was tap water, which had sufficient levels of chlorine and was not found to contain any enteric organisms. Water has the potential for nonpathogenic enteric organisms, as they survive for a much longer period than the enteric pathogens, especially *Salmonella* and *Shigella*.

As for the turtles, how do you examine them? Taking a swab culture of their shells would not be conclusive, as they swam in the contaminated water and would naturally be covered with the organisms present in it. No, a fecal or stool culture would be required. But turtles don't defecate in such a way that you can collect their stool intact from the environment. We determined that the best way would be to take rectal cultures. If you have ever held a turtle, you have observed that they pull in their necks, legs, and tails tightly to their bodies, and it is quite difficult to pull them out. But we did pull the tails out and gently inserted sterile swabs into the rectums of the turtles for culture. And they were positive for *Salmonella*.

At that time, these small turtles were popular pets, and there were no restrictions on the sale of them. Our findings were reported to the state and the Center for Disease Control, as it was known then. Similar reports popped up all over the country, and the CDC conducted investigations that ultimately led to strict regulations on the growth and intrastate transportation of turtles and reptiles. Now turtles must come from colonies that are determined to be free of *Salmonella.*

It is well understood that pathogenic organisms may be found in any animal and animal product or byproduct. Even under the most sanitary of conditions, contamination can enter. Virtually all animals have the notorious *E. coli* in extremely large numbers in their intestinal tracts (including humans), and this organism is generally of low pathogenicity and indicates the presence of fecal matter. Fortunately, they are easily killed by heat and disinfectants. Thorough cooking of meat will eliminate these organisms, and it is only foods that may be consumed raw that constitute the increased probability of infections. Such foods as lettuce and other field crops that can be contaminated by "night soil" or contaminated water should be washed with potable water before use. Eggs cooked properly will not be a problem, but raw eggs as in eggnog can potentially transmit salmonellosis. Cross-contamination of raw fluids to the cooked product, such as carrying a broiled steak from the outdoor grill to the table using the same platter used to carry it from kitchen to grill is a serious problem. Don't do it!

Although chickens may not frequently harbor *Salmonella*, a very high percentage of fresh chicken carcasses in the general meat market or food store will have the enteric pathogen *Campylobacter jejuni* and related species. This organism was not even known years ago, and yet it is now not unusual as the cause of diarrhea, but it, too, is easily killed by heat.

There is one species, *Salmonella pullorum*, that causes white diarrhea in chickens and can infect humans. Flocks of chickens, especially laying hens, need to be certified as pullorum free.

CHAPTER 7

# Leprosy in Paraguay

THE SUMMER I FINISHED MY master's degree at the University of Tennessee, Knoxville, I was selected to go to the Hospital Bautista in Asuncion, Paraguay, as a student summer missionary with the Southern Baptist Convention. In fact, on the day of commencement, I took a flight from Knoxville to Miami, Florida, to meet a nurse from Texas and to commence our trip to Paraguay. She was also a student summer missionary. We did not take a direct flight but were sent around South America to visit other mission sites and then were to report back to our respective campuses upon our return. Our trip took us to Cuba, (Castro had just taken control.) Panama, Ecuador, Peru, Chile, Argentina, and then Paraguay. On my return I also stopped in Brazil and Venezuela.

In Paraguay, my job was to review the existing microbiology procedures and techniques and to improve and extend them if possible. The Hospital Bautista was a mission staffed with missionary doctors and nurses as well as national workers. It had a nursing school with students from a number of countries throughout South America. I was given a room in one of the doctor's residence on the campus of the hospital. The hospital grounds comprised the hospital, three residences, the nursing school, and the residence hall for the student nurses. Two missionary nurses lived in an apartment building across the street. This hospital was one of the best, if not the best hospital in Paraguay. At that time (1959) in much of South America, nursing care was not provided twenty-four hours a day. Usually, the nurses and aides left in the evening and returned in the morning, but not at the Hospital Bautista, where round-the-clock care was provided.

Paraguay is a very interesting country. There are four languages in common use: Spanish, Guarani, English, and German. Guarani is a native language spoken by many people in Paraguay and surrounding countries. Many German-speaking people migrated there after both World War I and World War II and most lived in the Chaco area in the northern part of Paraguay. It was widely held that many Germans there were Nazis or sympathizers, and some still wore swastikas. But there were also many German Mennonites and Mennonites from Canada living on large farms throughout the country.

In our laboratory, the technologists spoke one language well and a second one to some degree and could communicate well within the lab and with any client or patient who might come for testing. In my case, I had completed two years of German while at the University of Kentucky and could understand more than I could speak. The lab was directed by a "doctor" who was a biochemist. He was only there part-time and owned a private lab and pharmacy. The regulations are quite different than here in the United States. Pharmacies are not controlled by the government but are owned by pharmacists or just about anyone who has some knowledge of the field of pharmacy. A physician's prescription was not always necessary. Anyone who has completed what we would call a bachelor's degree is called "doctor," so that is what I was called, too, even though I only had my master's degree.

At that time, Latin America shut down each day at 1:00 p.m. for a two-hour siesta. Just about everything was closed for this time, and most people stopped work and took a nap. This was difficult for me, as I had never done it before. The hospital still maintained nursing staff on duty during the siesta, but everything else was closed. This meant that the day was extended into the evening a little, and most Paraguayans didn't eat their evening meal until 7:00 p.m. or later. Then the people flooded the streets, with the single ladies standing in small groups on street corners under the lights while the men roamed around, met friends, and socialized. There were not nearly as many street lights as in an American city, and the ones that were there were not too bright. Throughout the land, especially on the outskirts of the city and in the countryside, it seemed that anyone who owned a radio was playing it at full volume. During the night, the radios were off, but the country had many flocks of chickens, and the roosters crowed all night long and not just at dawn. It took one some time to adjust to these changes in environment.

The hospital also was a teaching hospital for physicians, and it had a nursing school. There were both medical and surgical residents. The goal of many of these residents was to qualify for additional training in the United States, and as required by the Paraguayan government, they had to be able to speak English. Therefore, many took the opportunity to speak to me to practice their English.

The lab had some unusual difficulties in microbiology. There was no source of powdered agar, which is the substance required to make solid media for the growth of microorganisms. Agar is made from the seaweed *Agar-agar*, which has been used for many years in the food industry. What we had were large pieces of the dried seaweed, which we had to pulverize to make the powdered agar. Much of the dehydrated commercial media they had was old and had solidified in the jars. In order to make media, I reconstituted the solid media by dissolving it, redrying it, and then grinding it to a powder. It did make passable media. We also used human blood, although this is not usually recommended for several reasons. We would use outdated blood from the blood bank, and one of us would "volunteer" to donate blood if required.

In addition, the hospital where the physicians would work in the emergency room and in clinics and see private patients, the two American missionary physicians also worked on the weekends with one of the Baptist churches or mission outreach programs. One was a pediatrician and the other a thoracic surgeon. The pediatrician worked with the church he and his family attended and would also visit a clinic out in the jungle area of eastern Paraguay monthly. I eagerly accepted his invitation to go there with him.

On the way to this clinic, we would pass a leper colony. There are many thousands of lepers in tropical South America, most of whom can be maintained on the required medicines in their own homes. But this colony had been in existence for many years, and a doctor with another mission group was in residence there. Whenever Dr. Skinner came by, he would stop for a short visit, and they could exchange information and bring supplies in whenever needed and available. I must admit I had trepidation going into the colony. But leprosy is not highly contagious and still not well understood. We walked through the colony, and I saw a great many afflicted people. One couple was of particular interest. They were very short Guarani natives and had met, fallen in love, and married while in the colony. They had several children. None of the children showed any symptoms of the disease.

We traveled farther up the road and pulled over at a spot along the highway. The clinic was seven or more kilometers down a trail through the jungle to the village of the Indians. This tribe was semicivilized by our standards; they wore only breechcloths or skirts. The little boys ran around naked (thus showing they were male, a source of pride to the tribe), whereas the little girls wore grass skirts. They lived in mud-walled huts with palm-leaf roofs. The ground around the front was packed-down red soil, and a cooking fire was maintained in this front yard. The yards as well as the houses were swept several times a day with grass brooms.

The day we arrived was hotter than normal. When we got out of our car and started unloading the bags of supplies and medicine, the guides from the village were there, but the horses we expected to ride to the village weren't. It was, they explained, too hot for the horses. Therefore, we had to walk to the village, but the men did grab the bags and carried them for us.

Arriving in the small village, Dr. Skinner set up his clinic under the porch of one of the huts. There was no privacy. As he examined each patient, all the rest of the villagers stood around and watched. He needed an interpreter to help, as many did not speak Spanish, and Dr. Skinner had not yet learned enough Guarani. He would write down the patient's name, diagnosis, the medicine he was giving him or her, and the instructions on how the patient was to take it. If he had it in the bags we had brought to the village, he would give it to the patient right there, but there were a few patients for whom he had medicine in the station wagon out on the main road. Some of the villagers would go with us and bring back those medicines.

But one patient was treated somewhat differently. As with each patient, the doctor took his history. His story was that he had knelt by his cooking fire; noticed the smell of burning flesh; and, looking down, discovered he was kneeling on a red-hot coal. It had burned through his skin, and he had not even felt the pain. Dr. Skinner examined the hole and cleaned it out. Taking a pin, he then stuck it into the man's skin near the lesion. A faint red circle was visible a few millimeters around the lesion. When the pin was stuck into the skin outside that line, the patient jumped with pain, but he had no reaction when the pin was stuck into the skin inside the ring. Dr. Skinner shook his head. He explained to the patient that he was not sure what the exact problem was. He wanted him to go to the nearest hospital for further examination, and that would be at the leper colony we had visited. Would that be OK? The patient agreed. He was given an antibiotic ointment to put in the hole to stop local infection and went away happy.

After all the patients were seen and treated, it was time to hold the evening service, as it was Sunday. The villagers had songbooks and a leader and had begun the service singing at another larger hut close by. Dr. Skinner was to preach, and the leaders led him over to the front of the group. I tagged along and stopped at the rear of the group. As they were singing, a younger woman saw me and thought I'd like to share the hymnal she was holding. She came over and extended her hand with the book to me. Of course, I had to stand close enough to share it with her. Did I mention the women are topless? Have you ever sung a hymn of the church with a bare breast hanging over the hymnal? Especially for a young man not used to seeing such a sight, it was most difficult. Dr. Skinner was happy to relate my discomfiture when we got back home. But I digress.

It was getting dark when we were ready to leave. It had cooled somewhat, so the horse was available and needed to bring the guide back through the dark jungle. Several men started out with me ahead of Dr. Skinner, as he needed to leave the instructions. We hurried along as it gets dark fast in the jungle, and there were dangerous animals. (Including large snakes—one of the nurses had visited the clinical previously and tripped over one of the large boa constrictors crawling across the path.)

We were perhaps halfway to the road when we heard the sound of a galloping horse, turned to see a riderless horse tearing up the path toward us. The men tried to grab the reins and succeeded in finally catching and calming it down. Where was Dr. Skinner? Was he OK? We started back up the path and found him, unhurt, embarrassed but smiling as he related how he had been thrown off. But he gamely remounted the horse and went on ahead. It was dark when we got to the road, but nothing else untoward happened. Dr. Skinner had all the things he needed in order and gave them to the guide who mounted up and headed back to the village, and we got started back to Asuncion.

As we rode along, Dr. Skinner first related all the cases to me and chided me about the hymn sing. Then he asked me, "What do you think the man I sent up to the colony had? Did you think I really didn't know the diagnosis?"

I said I thought he had another reason but knew the diagnosis. I didn't.

He laughed. "It is leprosy. I didn't want to tell him that, as the villagers would have thrown him out of the village and not let him back. He can be seen by Dr. Smith, and he'll put him on the right medications and not give the stigma of being a leper. In that village, it would not be accepted."

That was the first time I saw a case of leprosy diagnosed. There are two types: one is disfiguring with lumpy wart-like growths, and the second is anesthetic—killing off the nerves. And obviously, the man had the second type.

Sometime later, I was working in the lab, and someone came and asked for me. Dr. Skinner wanted to see me in his office. When I arrived there, he was seated and talking to a young woman who was rather attractive except for one thing, which Dr. Skinner pointed out to me. Near the tip of her nose was a wart-like growth. Then he took a sterile swab and rubbed the inside of each naris, put the swab into a tube, and handed it to me. "Here. Go do an acid-fast stain on this ASAP."

I did, and to my surprise, I saw a few thin, slightly curved acid-fast rods and went back to tell Dr. Skinner. He smiled and told me that was diagnostic of leprosy. The easiest way they had to find this was the acid-fast stain, as the leprosy pathogen cannot be grown by routine culture, although it has been grown in the footpads of mice and in armadillos. This was the lepromatous type, and so I saw my second diagnosis of leprosy.

Years later, I specialized in mycobacterial diseases and mycology and ran the special lab in a major teaching hospital, but I never saw another case of leprosy. Once I was invited to give a lecture on mycobacterial diseases to the students at Tufts Medical School, which I was pleased to do. I included in my lecture the reason the Bible gives instructions to those who recover from leprosy that they are to return to the priests for examination. If the priests determined the leprosy was "cured," the person was deemed clean and could return to his or her home. Now leprosy wasn't curable in biblical times, so what constituted being cured? The word "leper" can mean "foul" and/or "loathsome," and I said that to an outburst of laughter. All heads turned toward a red-faced student seated high up in the lecture hall. After the lecture concluded, someone informed me that the student's surname was Leper. My turn to be embarrassed, and I didn't get the chance to apologize. Names can sometimes lead to such situations, but one can't help what names mean.

## CHAPTER 8

# Return to Paraguay

A FEW YEARS AFTER MY first visit to Paraguay, I got the urge to return. I was then working in Boston and would need to take a leave of absence so I could go and have a job when I returned. I first needed to see if that would be possible. I requested a three-month leave, which was granted. I then contacted the Hospital Bautista in Asuncion and found out the same physicians were still there and would be happy to have me return. I made the arrangements and asked the missionaries if there was anything they did not have that I might be able to bring them. They did not have the necessary instrument to run sodium and potassium testing: a flame photometer. I could locate and acquire a basic instrument but, of course, without the tanks of gas needed to run it. The missionary, Dr. Skinner, told me if I could bring it down as carry-on luggage, we would probably be able to bring it into the country without going through customs. It was not that big, so I could carry it on and, if necessary, keep it on my lap or on the floor at my feet. I went down for what was the winter season up north and flew from Boston to Asuncion.

The flight left on time without any trouble. I had no problems with my luggage including the unusual carry-on. I seriously doubt if I would be able to do it now, with the post 9/11 regulations. The flight was supposed to be nonstop, but somewhere between New York and Puerto Rico, we ran into trouble. One of the engines developed problems and burst into flames. They were extinguished, but we lost use of the engine. The pilot informed us we would need to land in San Juan for repairs. To effect a safe landing, the opposite engine would be shut down, and we would land with two engines. I did not think anything of it at the time until, as we were making our final approach, we were instructed to put our heads in our laps and clasp our knees for a possible crash landing. Even that didn't excite me as much as when, after we had touched down on the runway, I looked out the window to see many fire engines and other trucks racing along beside us. The pilot laid on the brakes and reversed the two remaining engines, and we roared to a stop just feet short of the end barriers. In fact, they had to pull us back and turn us around to continue taxiing to the terminal.

There were more problems. The engine could not be repaired, and we had to change airplanes to continue our flight. But there were fewer first-class seats on the second plane, and a fight broke about over which passengers would give up their first-class status to join us in the poorer section. Didn't they realize we had come very close to a crash landing? Some people!

The continuation flight was without incident. Upon arrival, I grabbed my briefcase, put it on top of the instrument, and proceeded off the plane. As I came into the customs area, Dr. Skinner greeted me from beyond the first barrier, but he was able to come through and join me as the young customs officer began examining my luggage. Since I still knew very little Spanish, I was happy when Dr. Skinner volunteered to answer and/or interpret for me. Everything was fine with my passport and visa, but the instrument became a point of contention. If it was a new instrument, it should be admitted through customs and taxed. At that time, it might be taxed at more than 1,000 percent of its stated value. Dr. Skinner made the arguments that (1) it was my personal property, (2) I had carried it off with me, (3) it was used, and (4) it was a gift to the hospital and the country.

The official had a problem. He knew he should really hold the instrument for customs and the taxes, but he also needed to see a good doctor. In Paraguay at that time, people could only go to a medical facility in the area where they lived. The Hospital Bautista was generally known to be the best in the country, but he did not live in the area served by it. Did Dr. Skinner know if there was a way he could come and see him personally? Dr. Skinner thought the official could very easily come and see him in his office at the hospital the next week. A smile crossed the face of the official, the rubber stamp came down and I, with the flame photometer, entered the country.

I soon got into a routine, working at the hospital and being involved in the activities of the missionaries, too. There was one surprise awaiting me, though. One of the doctors led me back to the kitchen, and there was a dietician from the United States whom I had met before when both of us were in the wedding of mutual friends.

Problems arose, however. One was with the flame photometer. The bio-chemist didn't know how to run it, and we had to get the instructions translated and arrange to get the tanks of gas. Air and propane were required. These never arrived while I was there, and after I was back in Massachusetts, I learned the biochemist had obtained and hooked up a tank of oxygen instead of the clearly marked air, and when he ignited the gas mixture, the machine blew up and was destroyed. Fortunately, no one was injured.

A second problem was getting a badly needed x-ray machine out of customs. Paraguayan officials had assessed the machine with many taxes and duties, far more than the hospital could afford and many times more than the value of the machine. It was a real shame, as it was for the use of the hospital and the care of the Paraguayan people and not for a profit-making organization. One of the physicians was working hard to see if he could get most of these fees, if not all of them, removed, and he hit on an interesting idea. He knew I had specialized in diagnosing tuberculosis, related diseases, and fungal diseases. He also had learned the Paraguayans had a national laboratory that could use some help in that area. He offered my services to them with my knowledge and agreement. They accepted and arranged for me to work there three or four days a week. They sent a driver in an old, small pickup truck every morning, and he returned me to the Hospital Bautista after noon. The labs only worked until siesta time and then closed for the day.

There were two ladies working in the TB section of the lab. Neither had any formal education, but they had been trained to process specimens, prepare and read cultures, and stain the specimens and positive cultures. The country was very poor and the equipment old, including such things as hand-cranked centrifuges. They made their own media, and many of the metal-topped tubes were rusted and had holes in them, not a very good situation. The ladies were not too happy to see me there. The "doctors" overseeing the lab didn't do any of the testing they just reviewed the results.

One of the things I noticed was they did not concentrate specimens and therefore only did smears on direct specimens. With the doctor's permission, I wrote up instructions on preparing concentrates and modified the staining procedure they used. These required translation into Spanish, and the ladies rather reluctantly began to follow them, and I, as tactfully as I could, directed them. It wasn't until one day that I got out of my chauffeur-driven truck and was greeted by the two of them coming to meet me, smiles on their brown faces. "*Frotis, frotis,*" one said, waving a glass slide. I took it, went in, and put it under the microscope. There were the nice red curving rods typical of mycobacteria. It was the first positive slide with the concentrated method, on a sample that had been negative with the direct method they were using before—a success. Thereafter, I had no trouble with suggestions I made for improving the lab.

For almost three months I went there. It was good for me, too. There are many parasites in the tropics, and the lab diagnosing them was next to the TB lab. I would go there frequently to see positive specimens. The scientist who had devised the means of using the "kissing beetle" to feed on patients, wait for several days, and then examine the intestinal contents for the trypanosomes worked there. (Reading blood smears for malaria here and a three-week vacation I spent in Columbia reading malarial smears and examining stools for parasites gave me great experience and training for subsequent work throughout my career.)

The payoff came later. Our surgeon met with the Paraguayan treasurer and customs officials regarding the x-ray machine and mentioned how I was helping them in the laboratory without any payment or salary of any kind. Eventually, almost all the fees and taxes were removed, and the machine was released from customs. (That, too, happened after I was gone, so I never got to see it in operation. Some things move rather slowly there.)

During this visit, I stayed in the call room at the hospital. If a woman was in labor and the ob-gyn needed a place to sleep waiting for the time of delivery, that was where he would stay. There were two double bunks, and I slept in one. It was rare to have someone else there, but when it happened, I was invited to go along and observe the delivery or an emergency surgery, which happened several times. When I could be of use, I would scrub in and go into the surgical suite. One night, a British man who owned a cattle ranch in Paraguay was brought in. He had fired an employee who came back later, called the man out into the street old-West style, and then shot him five times with a .22 pistol. I helped by holding his side open while the surgical staff sewed up the internal wounds. He survived the surgery well but later developed complications they were unable to treat with what they had there, and he eventually died. Although every surgical precaution was observed, the surgical suites were not air-conditioned, so the "windows" (there were no glass panes) were open for a cooling breeze, if possible.

In one case the surgeon drilled four burr holes in a young girl's skull as I watched from behind. After the fourth hole was completed, he inserted a long needle attached to a large syringe and, pulling back gently, aspirated perhaps ten cubic centimeters of pus. He pushed it out into a sterile tube, handed it to me, and instructed me to go and Gram-stain it and see what I could find. It was positive for chains of gram-positive cocci. We did not have anaerobic culture methods, and it did not grow on the aerobic culture plates. Antibiotics were selected for the gram-positive cocci and possible anaerobes, and the girl recovered nicely.

Most of the other stories I could tell would not be within the scope of this book, but it was a good experience for me and helped me in my career in many ways.

## CHAPTER 9

# Barber's Itch

BARBER'S ITCH IS A DISEASE of the past, at least in this country. It is reminiscent of the days when a man would go to his local barber shop for a shave, before there were disposable razors, or the razors would be disinfected before use on the next man. Barber's itch is a fungal disease of the skin on one's face and is transmitted from person to person, usually by the gentle art of the shave. Of course, there must have been a first case, and where it came from would be difficult to determine. We would not expect to have seen it in a hospital setting as, at least in the "olden days," it would have been diagnosed and treated by the local family doctor.

But the case that we saw did not come to us in that manner. If a patient is admitted to the hospital with an infectious disease, he or she will generally be placed in isolation specific to the type of infection the patient has. Such cases are reported to the infection-control coordinator (nurse) for verification and follow-up. In the hospital in which I was working at the time, I was training a nurse in the practice of infection control, since the hospital had recently instituted the position. She reported to me that the hospital had admitted a young man with a severe case of boils in his beard, and he was in contact isolation. This meant anyone going into the room would be required to put on full garb: gown, mask, hat, gloves, and bootees. The patient would have to gown up and put on a mask if leaving the room for any reason. The causative agent for boils is almost always *Staphylococcus aureus*, and staph infections are always isolated until the patient is free of the organism.

Since the patient had been admitted with the diagnosis, we did not have an isolate in the lab for further work such as antibiotic susceptibility testing. Repeat cultures were taken, and to our surprise, we did not grow out the staph. We knew the patient had not been receiving antibiotics long enough to render the boils sterile. I called the physician who had admitted the patient and asked if he had obtained a culture previously or had only acted on the appearance of the boils and the usually suspected agent (goes to the adage "when you hear hoofbeats, think horses not zebras"). As it turned out, the physician had a small laboratory in his office and did culture some specimens such as throat, nose, and superficial wounds—a not entirely unusual practice, but one I do not recommend, as there are many controls and conditions laboratories such as ours are required to do for certification that office labs do not perform. Also, I learned that the vendors of culture media charged the physicians much more per culture plate than what we had to pay. (At that time, some doctors paid five dollars for blood agar plates, whereas we paid less than one dollar because of the great difference in quantities used.)

I explained that we would like to do the susceptibility testing and phage-type the organism to compare it with isolates we maintained in the lab that were isolated within the hospital. He thought he had the culture plate there and would gladly bring it in to me when he came to check on his patient. And he did. We were quite surprised that the culture plate had only a few scattered colonies, and these were not of *S. aureus* but the closely related and generally nonpathogenic species *Staphylococcus epidermidis* (coagulase negative). *S. epidermidis* can cause infections under certain circumstances especially if a patient is immunocompromised. It seemed probably to us that the "boils" were not boils but some other condition, but what?

I obtained permission from the patient's physician to try to determine what was going on after I reported our results to him. When I visited the patient's room, there were several family members sitting in his room, fully garbed as required. They were very concerned that they would also come down with the infection and transmit it to others. He was, I learned, a teacher in a high school in a small town not too far from us. There was concern his students might have been exposed and were in danger of picking up the infection also. I also learned that he had been taken to surgery that morning and had thirteen of the boils lanced and drained. I set up cultures on some of these, which again did not grow staph.

The patient had a full beard except for under his chin and on his neck area. Most of the boils were in the beard area, but some were obvious on his neck. I asked him how much the boils hurt; he said they did not hurt except the ones that had been lanced. With permission, I gently squeezed several with my gloved hand, and he did not flinch. Now, if you've ever had a boil or carbuncle, you know they are quite painful. To me, these were not boils. I was not certain at the time exactly what they were, but I had an idea. Retreating to my office, I went through several books and atlases until I found what I thought might be the case: *Tinea barbae.*

With this in mind, I located the family physician and presented my idea to him. He took the thought in mind and went to his office. I received a call a little later, and he was somewhat chagrined. He had been trained in Germany years ago, and when he recalled his experience there and saw the pictures of *Tinea barbae*, he recognized it was probably that.

Meanwhile, we kept the blood plates and examined them daily. There, along the lines of inoculation, very small, fuzzy colonies characteristic of fungi had appeared. These were slow-growing colonies, and it took several days before we could examine them microscopically and recognize the characteristic of a dermatophyte. We had the infectious agent, and it did not require either hospitalization or isolation of the patient. Additionally, the patient had complained that he now had several round, red lesions on his shoulder he did not have when he came in. I examined them, and they appeared characteristic of the notorious ringworm (which is not a worm). I obtained skin scrapings of the edges of the lesion. Upon microscopic examination, the thin hyphae characteristic of a dermatophyte were observed.

The patient was put on antifungal therapy and sent home, much relieved he did not have an infection endangering his family or his students.

We were curious about the source of the organism. The patient had not gone to a barber shop and only used his own razor to shave his neck. But he was a farmer; it was winter, and he raised calves from his dairy herd. These young calves were kept indoors and were not exposed to the sun, which is lethal to some fungi. He told me many of these calves had lesions over much of their bodies, and these proved to be caused by dermatophytes also. The isolate we obtained from this patient was a species that consistently causes infections in cattle and other fur-bearing animals as well as humans.

Putting this all together, we concluded that he had gotten his organism from the calves and, by scratching his beard, had inoculated the spores into his skin. Shaving helped spread it. This is an easily treated condition, and by spring he was again lesion free, and we had resolved another good case.

CHAPTER 10

# Atypical or Anonymous Mycobacteria

WHILE I WAS ATTENDING A national convention of the Society of American Microbiologists, I met a fellow former graduate student who introduced me to a couple of microbiology technologists from Boston. Because of that encounter, I was invited to come to Boston and interview for a position at one of the major teaching hospitals. I did so and learned from the director of the lab that he was planning on expanding it by upgrading the area of mycology and mycobacteriology (i.e., fungus and TB and TB-related organisms). I had been working with fungus cultures for some time but had little knowledge beyond what I'd had in my undergraduate training related to tuberculosis. That was fine with him, as he was willing to send me to the National Jewish Hospital in Denver, Colorado, for specific training in that area. I wanted to go back home and think it over, but he said he needed to know right then, so I agreed to take the position, fully thinking I could call back from Michigan and turn it down later. (I wanted to stay in Michigan, but the salary and potential were better in Boston. The company I worked for in Michigan wouldn't match the salary offered, so I left.)

After moving to Boston and starting to develop my section I did, indeed, go to Denver and spent two weeks learning the advanced procedures I needed to know. I also was introduced to a complete area of species of *Mycobacteria* with which I was not familiar. In fact, several of these were called anonymous, atypical, or mycobacteria other than TB (MOTT). The

53

research scientist there had been developing a serologic method of comparing these isolates. There are a few species that are well characterized and known to be nonpathogenic. Some are of low pathogenicity to humans or cause disease in animals other than humans or rarely in humans. One of these, *Mycobacterium bovis*, produces disease in cattle, deer, and related animals and has caused disease in humans. In fact, this is the organism for which pasteurization of cow's milk was developed. It is also the organism that makes the news when found in deer and is referred to as tuberculosis rather than bovine tuberculosis, as is presently found in the northeastern counties of lower Michigan. It is quite different, especially in means of transmission, in response to antibiotics, and in its appearance growing on culture media. *M. tuberculosis* (MTB) grows as raised, rough, cauliflower-like beige colonies, whereas most of the atypical organisms are smooth, softer appearing, and range in color from cream to yellow to bright orange. These latter isolates have often been ignored in the clinical laboratory and discarded. It is these organisms that I was taught to recognize and to follow up in my laboratory. Subsequently, more and more of these isolates have been proven to be the cause of a patient's disease. When the causative agent is properly recognized and identified, the patient can be treated with commonly used antibiotics, and a cure results. In this chapter, I shall relate some experiences with this group of organisms.

Tuberculosis is still one of the most common diseases throughout the world, although it has greatly been reduced here in the United States. In recent times, almost half of the new cases recognized each year in the United States are found in immigrants. In the early years of the last century, immigrants were checked for active TB and, if it was present, were sent back home. This is no longer true. This may also be responsible for the increase in multiple-resistant strains of *M. tuberculosis* being found and reported in the United States.

As with so many of the previously common infectious diseases, an effort has been made to develop a vaccine for tuberculosis. It has been a difficult task, as MTB has a chemical composition not readily given to produce adequate immune response. Using *M. tuberculosis* is not feasible, but the related *M. bovis*, especially an attenuated (weakened) strain called BCG, may be. As with any vaccine, it must be field tested once it has been demonstrated not to cause disease, serious side effects, or local reactions and yet to protect the patient. Before I talk about this further, I need to give you some more background on the MOTT group of organisms.

Dr. Ernest Runyon developed a scheme for the identification of these anonymous organisms so they could be at least grouped into recognizable related organisms. He had four groups, identified as Runyon groups I, II, III and IV. The one that was of most importance was group III, which came to be known as *M. bovis intracellulare*. Groups I through III were all slower-growing organisms, much like the notorious MTB, taking up to three weeks to appear on a culture slant. The group IV organisms are rapid growers, appearing in a little as two to three days, and a couple of them caused superficial skin lesions. Our job was to recognize these isolates, although we did not have all the procedures and means to identify them. For that purpose, we had to send them to the state department of health laboratory, which would, in turn and if required, send them on to the CDC laboratories in Georgia. (Eventually, our laboratory was sending more isolates on than all the rest of the labs in the state combined.) Because of this, we were very careful to examine and report the isolation of any species of acid-fast organism to the patient's physician for evaluation. In this manner we could diagnose and treat patients with some long-term conditions and subsequent cures.

Because of this background, we could recognize an unusual situation. Our institution had a branch in the state of Maine and worked closely with other clinics there. One of these had the privilege of working with the Micmac Native Americans who lived in northern Maine and in the adjacent parts of Canada. This population, unfortunately, had a high incidence of tuberculosis and became a natural site for the testing of the new vaccine developed from BCG. By vaccinating a large part of the population and comparing these patients with the part of the population not vaccinated, the efficacy of the vaccine could be determined. (This was also being done in Haiti.) During the time of this trial, several patients arrived at the clinic serving the Micmac population with draining lesions at the site of the vaccination. Routine cultures of these lesions failed to show growth, and treatment with antibiotics failed to cure them. Additional material was obtained from these lesions and sent to our laboratory for complete culture evaluation including routine, fungal, and mycobacteria. The routine cultures failed to show any significant growth, as did the fungal cultures. However, the initial acid-fast stain (the method used in our laboratory at the time was the Ziehl-Neelsen stain, which was standard for acid-fast organisms) was positive for thin, straight acid-fast rods. The cultures became positive for smooth, yellowish, butyrous colonies. This was consistent with Runyon group III and with the BCG organism. We did not have the methods necessary for identification, and therefore sent it to the state laboratory. They forwarded it on to the CDC, which subsequently identified it as BCG and directly connected it with the vaccine used. So it became evident that a case of local infection was a rare but possible side effect of the vaccine for tuberculosis.

Years later, I was working in a hospital back in Michigan when a patient came in to see me with a referral and request for evaluation of a lesion on his forearm. His physician and I had connected previously on a case of sporotrichosis (reported in chapter 3), and he felt I might have some suggestion about this lesion, as it was not responding to his treatment. As was usual in such cases, I ran a full panel of cultures except for viral. This would be routine, fungal, and acid-fast. The initial bacterial Gram stain and culture were negative. A subsequent review of the Gram stain did show faintly staining gram-positive rods. Fungal examinations were negative. The acid-fast stain was positive for acid-fast rods, but the cultures were not positive in the first couple of days. I contacted the physician to learn more about the history of the case. The patient was employed at a local nursing home and had received the required annual skin test for tuberculosis. We contacted the nursing home and found there were several additional cases of infectious-appearing lesions at the site of the skin test.

After several more days, the acid-fast culture began to show several small colonies that were smooth, pale yellow, and, when tested, positive for acid-fast rods. They appeared to me to be a Runyon group III or related organism and reminded me of the cultures obtained from the Micmac Native Americans. Since we did not have methods for identification, the culture was submitted to the state health department laboratories. Later, I received word from them that the culture was not to be identified. The lab felt it was a nonpathogenic species, and they were concentrating on the MTB strains. I raised objections to this and requested the isolates be sent to the CDC, based on my previous experience. This was done, and the CDC identified the isolate as consistent with BCG.

This caused quite a problem. How would several cases of local skin lesions be infected with BCG? The skin test was done with PPD, which is not a viable organism but the derivative of *M. tuberculosis* and would be sterile. It was necessary for the state to conduct a study of what was happening at the nursing home. It was found that all the patients and employees had been skin tested with the TB vaccine and not with the PPD skin test. Neither the nurse who administered the test nor the pharmacist who sent her the vials of vaccine had not noticed they were using the wrong material. The size of the vials and the color of the labels were the same. They had not read the labels. (I learned later that the nurse lost her license over the incident, but to my knowledge, nothing was done to the pharmacist.) At almost the same time, a similar occurrence was found in Ohio and both were reported in the Morbidity and Mortality Weekly Report (MMWR), although no reference was made to how we found it in Michigan. Subsequently, the color of the labels was changed and other alterations made to help those using the materials differentiate more easily. Fortunately, these lesions can be cured without much damage to the patient.

There are many isolates of acid-fast organisms that go unnoticed and untreated, as the isolates are not followed up or identified. There are several of the anonymous or MOTT species that are known to cause disease, and each need to be carefully evaluated, unlike isolates of MTB, which are always pathogenic and must be treated.

Once, when I was working in the TB lab I had set up, we received a very unusual specimen with the request to culture it for TB: a nose culture. At first I thought this must be someone's mistake, possibly in taking the specimen, (why not sputum?) or perhaps they had requested the wrong culture and really wanted us to culture the specimen for routine bacterial organisms. But upon checking with the floor, we were reassured that both the specimen and request were correct. It seemed this patient had some type of chronic disease, and so far he had progressed from his physician's office through several hospitals and finally to our institution, and a diagnosis had yet to be made. I did not find a specific procedure on how to process a nasal culture for mycobacteria, but I decided to process it in the original specimen tube as with a sputum specimen.

Perhaps I should explain to the reader the whys and wherefores of processing specimens for mycobacteria. If the request is made for a culture from a specimen that is normally sterile—for example, cerebral-spinal fluid or joint aspirates—there is no need to process the specimen, and it can be put onto media directly. However, if it is from a specimen such as sputum, then the usual microorganisms present will soon overgrow any mycobacteria present and many times completely digest the basal medium on which it is inoculated. To retrieve the mycobacteria that may be present, it is necessary to kill off the other bacteria present, and this was done by subjecting the specimen to a strong solution of sodium hydroxide for a period and then neutralizing the specimen back to a neutral pH. This is necessary as mycobacteria are also subject to the lethal effects of the sodium hydroxide but are much more resistant to it than other kinds of bacteria. It is a balancing act between killing off all bacteria and maintaining the mycobacteria present.

After processing the nose culture, we inoculated and incubated it in a special incubator that had more carbon dioxide than was found in the incubators for routine bacterial cultures. Each culture was examined on a weekly basis for up to ten weeks, as MTB may take that long to grow to a visible size. To our surprise, small colonies typical of MTB eventually appeared, and we took the required steps to identify the colonies—the niacin test being the most important one at the time. But this required a large amount of growth and took up to several weeks following the finding of the initial growth. Of course, the acid-fast stain was done. We observed acid-fast organisms typical of MTB and reported this to the physicians in charge of the patient. We immediately received several phone calls checking on the results and asking for identification and verification of the result. The idea that it could be tuberculosis was very low on their list of possible diagnoses. It proved to be *M. tuberculosis* and created a lot of excitement in the infectious-disease department. The patient was immediately placed on appropriate antibiotics for tuberculosis, and eventually, a cure was brought about.

In most teaching hospitals, there are rounds, which are presented frequently (usually every month) in all departments, and then grand rounds, which are presented for all the medical staff, in which the most troubling and interesting cases are given for the benefit of all, from the medical novice to the most senior physicians present. They are usually given as case histories, as the first doctor attending the patient would have found and presented at times to a visiting expert in the field of the department (e.g., infectious disease, orthopedic, surgery). The expert then questions the presenter and asks for the next steps taken, such as viewing the X-rays and lab results, and this continues until all information except the ultimate diagnosis is given, usually by the pathologist. The visiting physicians give their primary diagnosis and continue with a list of other diagnoses they would consider possible. In the clear majority of times, the visiting physician gets it right, but on very rare occasions, the correct diagnosis may not be given at all or may be way down on their list. Of course, if you did not get the diagnosis, you felt vindicated if the visiting expert was also stumped by the case.

The city I was in for this case has four medical schools, and there is an exchange between two in which every other Friday afternoon, we would have infectious-disease rounds at our institution and the alternate week at the other institution. The visiting physician coming to our medical center was considered the dean of infectious diseases in all New England and was known throughout the country. We always hoped the case that we would present to him would stump him or at least cause him some trouble. We thought this would be one such case, as it had taken months to find the correct diagnosis, so the room was filled with students, faculty, and staff. We presented the case, and we all sat there with great anticipation. Dr. W. asked three questions, but right now I only remember one: Was there bilateral rupture of the ear drums? And the presenter said yes. Dr. W. slapped his hand on the table. "Tuberculosis," he said, and many jaws dropped. In three questions he came up with the answer that had eluded so many for so long. He gave a little laugh. "You guys are too young," he said. "When tuberculosis was in its prime, we saw these cases all the time." It seems that a person with pulmonary TB coughs so much the sputum can get up the eustachian tubes and into the ear, and the resultant growth ruptures both ear drums.

Medical grand rounds, which are also presented monthly, are major conferences in which rare and unusual cases are presented. They are then published in a major medical journal. In Boston, these are held in the Ether Dome of the Bulfinch Building at Massachusetts General Hospital and are attended by the most senior and well-known physicians in town. Many times, the experts are visiting physicians from other medical schools throughout the country. The Bulfinch Building is one of the oldest hospitals in the United States designed by the famous architect Charles Bulfinch, who also designed the capitol building of the Commonwealth of Massachusetts. The building resembles a state house and has a dome like most capitols and it contains an amphitheater (the Ether Dome). It is the site where the first public demonstration of the use of ether as an anesthetic agent was done. The dome is like a theater, with very steep rows of chairs facing a stage from which the case is presented, sometimes with the patient present, perhaps to be examined physically as well as orally. The senior staff who are present may ask questions, and the visiting physicians bring photographic and sometimes microscopic slides for viewing.

I went to these quite frequently and was involved with two of the cases, one with prior knowledge and one that was sprung on me unawares.

In the first case, we had made possible the diagnosis of tuberculous meningitis for the physician by finding a single acid-fast organism on a concentrated acid-fast smear of spinal fluid. Subsequently, the organism was isolated and identified, and the patient appropriately treated. Since this diagnosis was and is extremely rare, many of the physicians would have never seen such a case and most would never again, so it was selected for medical grand rounds. The presenter was a member of the infectious-disease faculty at Massachusetts General Hospital, and he had requested that we bring a microscope with the organism for the viewing of those present. My boss asked me to come to the rounds, sit in the wings of the stage, and make certain the slide was showing the acid-fast rod. He told me to check it after every three or four viewers.

It was a very good case presentation and excited a lot of interest. When the diagnosis was presented and the physicians learned it had been made as a result of the smear, a line of physicians came up to the microscope, peered in, and turned around gravely shaking their heads. I would go up as often as possible and almost invariably had to adjust the microscope to bring back the organism. Only one physician, as I remember, looked, didn't see it, and asked me to find it for him. I suspect many of them didn't see it but didn't want to say so.

We found this one acid-fast rod as a result of a technique I had instituted for use with spinal fluid specimens. If you put CSF on a slide, it can spread in a large circle, thus diluting out the specimen. One method is to centrifuge a portion of the specimen and pour off the fluid, leaving a small amount of sediment in the bottom. This can then be placed on the slide effectively concentrating any organism or white blood cells present in the CSF. But this, too, may not be enough. What I did was to etch a ring on the slide with a diamond point pen, place a drop in the center, and let it dry. (Never use a wax pencil to form the ring; it interferes with the stain.) Then I added a second drop and let that dry, too. In this way I could add several more drops, thus concentrating much more CSF in a small area. This technique was published as a letter in a journal of infectious diseases.

The other case I'll present in chapter 15.

## CHAPTER 11

# Penicillin, Cheese, and Anaphylactic Shock

ONE OF THE BASIC, ESSENTIAL questions that must be asked of a patient is "Do you have any known allergies?" Without that knowledge, a patient could inadvertently be exposed to an allergen that could put him or her in a life-threatening condition known as anaphylactic shock. And if—potentially—a patient might be given an antibiotic, the specific question about allergies to antibiotics must be asked. Many people are allergic to such antibiotics as sulfa drugs and penicillin. What is not generally known is that penicillin is a derivative of the fungus *Penicillium notatum* and related species. Many people are probably familiar with the story of how Alexander Fleming discovered penicillin. (It is not unusual for a working microbiologist to see this phenomenon in his or her everyday work.) What may not be known is that some kinds of cheese, such as Roquefort and Camembert, are made by species of *Penicillium*. Roquefort is commonly known as blue or "blu" cheese, because of the blue-colored areas seen in the bricks of cheese. This color is because of the growth of the organism in the goat's milk used to make the cheese. When I learned this fact, my curiosity led me to obtain a good specimen of blue cheese, remove a small piece of the crumbly blue area, and examine it under the microscope. I was rewarded by seeing the typical hyphae and fruiting bodies of *Penicillium*. I also put pieces of the blue cheese onto cultures plates designed for the growth of fungi, and in a few days, small, white, fuzzy colonies appeared. After several more days of incubation, a typical blue-green color appeared, and the growth again demonstrated characteristic penicillia. I wished I had kept that culture as years later, we raised goats for the milk. (One of my sons was lactose intolerant, and cow's milk was a problem for him. Goat's milk was not.) I could have made my own Roquefort.

A byproduct of the growth is the production of raw penicillin. Cheese produced in the United States and perhaps in other countries as well is routinely pasteurized, and this process effectively eliminates the heat-sensitive raw penicillin. However, many of the foreign-made cheeses are not heat treated and may contain sufficient penicillin to elicit a significant response in a person sensitive to it. In some cases it can result in anaphylactic shock and possibly death. Whenever I lecture on this area of mycology—I taught a graduate-level course in medical mycology—I made a point of stressing this fact. Very frequently, I would have students in my class with known penicillin allergies but without knowledge of the cheese connection.

For a period at one teaching hospital, the residents in the infectious-disease department came to my laboratory for training in mycobacteriology and mycology. This time with me was optional, and some would spend only a little time, but others would make good use of it. I enjoyed showing the residents as much as I could during my time with them and made it a point to tell them about the cheese-penicillin connection.

One day as I was working, one of the residents who had recently spent time with me came running into my laboratory. "Quick, what is the cheese that contains penicillin?"

"Roquefort and Camembert, why?"

"Don't have time now. Will be back later." He ran out.

My curiosity piqued, I waited for his return, and return he did, not that day but a couple of days later. He strolled in casually and pulled up a chair. "Want to hear the story?"

"Of course."

"I'm working the emergency room now, and we had a patient brought in the other day in what appeared to be anaphylactic shock, but it could have been a number of other things. We learned he had been eating at Durgin-Park (a famous Boston restaurant) and was suddenly overcome with a choking feeling, rash, and fever. An ambulance was called, and he was brought here. We could learn from him that he hadn't any previous feeling of sickness that day, and it had come on suddenly as he was eating. One of the things he mentioned was salad, and I asked him what kind of dressing he had and learned it was Roquefort. Although I remembered you had told me some cheese and cheese-based dressings could have penicillin, I couldn't remember which. That's why I ran in here the other day. After learning that, we asked him about any allergies, and he was allergic to penicillin, and we concluded he was suffering anaphylactic shock. Also, I went down to Durgin-Park and checked out their source of cheese and learned they used only authentic imported French Roquefort cheese. Thanks."

Another case resolved satisfactorily, I might add.

Since that time and following my lectures, I have learned of several cases of reaction to eating cheese or dressing containing cheese but have been assured that most cheeses will have been heat treated and the penicillin destroyed. I must still conclude, however, that imported cheeses have the potential to contain penicillin, and a warning still must be given.

CHAPTER 12

# Whipped by a Rope: Pneumococcus

IT WAS A SIMPLE ACCIDENT. The workers were hauling building material from the ground to the second floor of the project using an old hemp rope-and-pulley system. When the rope was released, it whipped around, and the frayed end struck a worker in his face. Within a couple of days, his eye was red and swollen, and "matter"—pus—had formed in it, requiring a visit to his physician. His eye was cleaned and drops applied, but it didn't clear up the problem. Physical observation revealed the presence of scratch marks across the cornea and additional treatment began, probably some antibiotic, but which was unknown to us. When his eye continued to appear infected, the patient was sent to a special clinic dealing with eye, ear, and nose conditions. Cultures were taken, but no organism was isolated, and the eye continued to deteriorate. The patient was getting discouraged and, upon learning that his eye appeared to have a hazy or "fuzzy" growth at the edge of his cornea, decided to see another eye specialist in another hospital. He came across town to our institution.

The physician in our clinic carefully examined the patient's infected eye and felt certain it was an infectious agent, either bacterial or fungal. He called me to determine if there were any special techniques or procedures we might recommend. Our laboratory had been using "candle jars" for special cultures, such as cerebral-spinal fluid and respiratory specimens. This method is easy to implement: the culture plates are put into a large jar with a wide mouth (like a mayonnaise jar), and then a lighted candle is placed inside. As the candle burns, it uses up the oxygen, resulting in increased carbon dioxide. The jar lid is sealed with masking tape, and the jar is placed in the regular incubator.

(While this is a good method for routine use, it does not produce sufficient $CO_2$ for all organisms requiring it nor is it always controllable. Therefore, engineers designed an incubator into which carbon dioxide is piped from a tank to achieve 10 percent concentration and is monitored daily at the least. After placing culture plates in the incubator, the technologist presses a button to give an extra charge to replace the "spilled" carbon dioxide. Most routine bacteriology laboratories now use this type of incubator.)

Our discussion included how the specimen was collected and transmitted to the laboratory. It was possible a delay in the transmission could result in the death of microorganisms en route. Also, some types of swabs could be toxic to organisms. The physician was concerned that this delay might have been the reason the previous cultures had not shown significant growth. (That laboratory did not use candle jars.) He also requested that we culture the specimen for fungi as, the appearance of the lesion in the eye was that of a fungal colony. Although it is unusual, he proposed bringing the patient from his room to the lab, so I could obtain the culture and plate it directly and immediately. He would use a new platinum bacteriological loop to scrape the eye, and we would plate it out.

The doctor and patient arrived in due time. He was a vigorous young man but was nervous and anxious. I explained to him that anesthetic could be inhibitory to some organisms, and he agreed to tolerate a scraping with the sterilized loop. The physician gently scraped with the cooled loop and handed it to me to inoculate the plates: sheep blood agar and chocolate agar. Sabouraud was added for fungal organisms. The plates were immediately placed into a candle jar (except the Sabouraud plate).

But the physician was not satisfied with his first specimen. He placed several drops of anesthetic solution in the man's eye so he could scrape deeper and removed some of the cornea for a second set of plates. The cultures were placed in the incubator, and the patient returned to his room and the doctor to his office to await the results of the culture. We did not do a Gram stain, relying on the culture because of the small amount of inoculum available.

A fungus culture is held up to four weeks, and growth can appear at any time from a couple of days up to a month. Bacterial cultures will grow out overnight, although some kinds of bacteria may take several days.

The next morning, the plates were removed, and to our surprise, on the blood agar plate and the chocolate agar plate were small, wet, doughnut-like green colonies (alpha hemolytic). Further studies proved the isolate to be *Streptococcus pneumoniae*: the pneumococcus. But the question became why hadn't this organism been isolated in the previous cultures? Normally, the pneumococcus grows quite readily on blood and chocolate agar plates under the usual incubation conditions employed. After submitting this for pneumococcal typing and obtaining the results, we learned that this serotype was one known to have an absolute requirement for increased levels of carbon dioxide. The other laboratory had not used any method for providing the needed increase of $CO_2$.

The lungs expel more carbon dioxide than is present in ambient air and therefore provide the necessary carbon dioxide to organisms requiring it. But that did not explain nor could we come up with an explanation why this $CO_2$ strain of pneumococcus could grow in the eye and produce a lesion. We tested the isolate against several antibiotics by existing methods and it proved to be susceptible to tetracycline, which was used, and in a short time—days, not weeks—the patient's eye cleared up, and he could return to work.

There was no growth on the fungal cultures.

This is an example of how cooperation between the laboratory personnel and the medical staff can produce a satisfactory result. Also, it precludes jumping to conclusions. The appearance of the lesion in the eye was that of a fungal colony, not what would be expected of a bacterium.

It also was an example of the need to use better incubation conditions, which were available at the time but just not used (i.e., the lab had not kept up with advances in the field of microbiology). No matter how much experience one may have in a field, there is always room for improvement, and one should keep up with the literature and make changes.

CHAPTER 13

# Bread Mold and Diabetes: Phycomycoses

VIRTUALLY EVERYONE HAS OBSERVED GROWTH of a member of the family of phycomycetes. They are often referred to as bread molds and do commonly grow on bread as very loose, spider-web types of growth showing small black dots. (If you observe green growth tight to the surface of the bread, it is probably a member of *Penicillium* or *Aspergillus* species.) These organisms are ubiquitous but often prefer materials with large amounts of sugar and protein. It is sometimes difficult to initiate their growth on agar plates, but when they do grow, they can fill a plate in a couple of days and even lift the lid of the plate. The mycelia of these organisms are much wider than those of most fungal organisms, and some species do not have septa in the mycelium. Some produce roots, which help them anchor to a surface. They produce long fruiting bodies ending in round structures that fill with spores. The exact morphology of these fruiting bodies is useful in determining the genus of the organism. This structure eventually splits, and the spores are sprayed around their environment, are picked up in the air, and float around looking for a favorable place to land and sprout again. And sometimes this can be the human body in which, rarely, a resulting infection can lead to death.

Those of us who work in the clinical laboratory are rarely called to the morgue. Tissue specimens are collected there and taken in appropriate containers to the pathology laboratory. When indicated, the pathologist

69

may remove a portion of the specimen and forward it to the microbiology laboratory with requests for stains and cultures suggested by their trained observations. But there have been times when I have been asked to come to the morgue and give my opinion as to potential pathogens and/or get a specimen directly so there would be no delay in getting the microbiological studies initiated.

I was called to the morgue and asked to bring a sterile petri dish for a tissue specimen. The patient had been an African American man in late middle age who had bled to death from his nose and mouth. The underlying diagnosis was uncontrolled diabetes. He had extremely high levels of blood glucose, and his doctors were in the process of getting the diabetes under control. He had periods of unconsciousness and widely ranging levels of glucose when he suddenly began to bleed from his nose. They had used all means available to control the bleeding, but the rapid exsanguination had claimed his life. A postmortem had been ordered, and this included opening his cranium, removing the brain, and finding out what had occurred in his sinuses and frontal lobe. There were, of course, large clots of blood, but in probing these clots, it seemed as if they were being held together by some fibrous material or other matter that extended into the sinus cavities. The pathologist removed some of this material, put it into the sterile petri dish, and asked me to examine it microscopically as well as to set up all available cultures. In our laboratory at the time, this would include bacterial, fungal, and mycobacterial cultures but not viral. A portion of the material would be placed into a deep freeze to be held in case pathological examination indicated the possibility of viral infection.

Initial smears, which were stained by Gram's method, failed to show any bacteria. In specimens such as this, it was my policy to include direct microscopic examination. Small pieces of material were placed on a glass slide and a cover slip put on top and gently pushed down. (A hard push could result in the material flying off the slide and contaminating the surrounding area.) I had also developed the procedure using only sterile water or saline. A commonly requested procedure for examining material is the KOH preparation. For reasons I'll discuss in another section, I did not use KOH, except for examining hair, skin, or nail specimens. When I put the specimen from this man under the microscope lens and looked, I was surprised to find a tangled mass of very large fungal mycelia. These were also quite wide and resembled to us those of the phycomycetes. We reported this to the pathologist and began a literature search to see if this was the type of case from which a phycomycete would be isolated. It was. There are several genera of phycomycetes that have been isolated from humans including *Rhizopus*, *Mucor*, *Absidia* and *Cunninghamella*. It would be necessary to grow out the organism to specifically identify it, not that it would matter to this patient or to others, as the treatment would be the same regardless of the species. The biggest problem if a patient is infected is that the treatment for fungal organisms at that time was *Amphotericin B* ("Ampho terrible"). This is a toxic antifungal agent and must be given in a low concentration initially and the dose increased slowly day by day to build it up in the body to levels sufficient to kill the fungi before the level becomes toxic to the body. This works quite well for the usual slower-growing fungal agents, but the growth of the phycomycetes is so rapid it would overgrow the patient before the lethal levels could be reached. The cure required physically—surgically—removing the infected tissue.

The cultures did not grow on the media used to grow fungi even though everyone who examined the specimen agreed there were fungal mycelia present. The tissue sections had been submitted for pathologic examination including using a special stain for fungi. They were all positive for fungal elements. I was stymied. Why did the organism grow so rapidly in a patient's tissue but fail to grow in vitro? One aspect of the case was the clue needed: the patient's high glucose level. Even though it was tested in the blood, it is well known that the glucose level in the tissue being fed by blood would also be very high. But was that the factor required for growth on the agar plates? I was curious to know if there was any other material I could use to attempt to grow the fungi. I went to my biochemistry text and located a table showing the chemical composition of fruit, vegetables, meat, and tissues, as well as other food groups. I found out that bread and human tissue were very close in basic composition (i.e. protein, minerals, and carbohydrates). This gave me an idea. Why not sterilize some bread in a petri dish and inoculate it with small pieces of the specimen? This I did. In some of the plates, I also added some sterile milk as an added nutrient source. The inoculated plates were incubated, and we waited. It seemed logical, as the phycomycetes were, after all, known as bread molds.

After a couple of days, a fuzziness started developing out of the pieces of the inoculum. But we had to be patient to allow the growth to develop sufficiently so the fruiting bodies would develop. We were successful in that the organism did continue to grow, and when the small black dots appeared in the plates, a small portion was pulled off and placed into a drop of lactophenol cotton blue solution for microscopic examination. This is done as the solution not only enhances visualization of the organism but is also lethal to it. The examination was positive for a species of the genus *Mucor* and therefore, the diagnosis would be known as mucormycosis. Fortunately, such cases are rare.

This is an example of the danger of uncontrolled diabetes.

And the additional problem is that spores of these organisms are ubiquitous. You can take samples of dust from just about anywhere, place it on dampened bread, and wait to see the fungi start growing. But don't do it! You don't need to enhance their presence.

Years later we were confronted by another case. A thirteen-year-old girl was admitted for acute appendicitis. The appendix was removed surgically, but a few days later, the wound was failing to heal and showed signs of infection. Routine cultures taken from the site failed to show significant growth. One of the factors under consideration for the lack of healing was the fact the patient was diabetic and was shown to have very high levels of glucose. One of the physicians attending her came to my laboratory to ask about the cause of black discoloration of the tissues around the surgical wound. The cause could have been a strain of pseudomonads, a rare species of anaerobes, and the phycomycetes. I asked if he could remove a small specimen of the tissue in the blackened area, and he complied with my request. Remembering the prior case gave me the idea of checking out the tissue by direct examination, which I did. A piece of the tissue was placed in a drop of the lactophenol cotton blue and teased apart by means of sterile dissecting needles as the tissue—mostly skin—was quite thick. After placing a cover slip on the specimen, I examined it under low (one hundred times) magnification, found the wide mycelia characteristic of the phycomycetes, and so informed the physician.

They were confronted with the problem of the necessity of treating the patient with the amphotericin B and controlling the diabetes. Again, we knew the organism could grow faster than we could get the levels of amphotericin B high enough to kill the fungus. The black ring around the wound seemed to be radiating out at a rapid clip, so the physician marked the location of the ring with a black marking pen. Then as time passed he came back and measured the progress of the ring through the skin layer in millimeters per hour. And it was a very high rate. The physician decided to surgically remove the tissue, cutting it at some distance in front of the progressing black line and for the full skin thickness. This specimen was also submitted for culture as well as the normal pathologic examination plus a special stain for fungal organisms. In all specimens, the fungal elements were found. In this case growth did appear on the routine fungal medium because we placed a drop of sterile 20 percent glucose on the plate to increase the concentration in the medium. It proved to be a species of phycomycete, but I don't remember exactly which one it was. For the first couple of days, the patient appeared to improve, and the wound edges were closed and appeared to be healing. But unfortunately, in another couple of days, some black areas again appeared and continued to grow rapidly across her abdomen. These areas were again shown to be fungal growth. The physician decided to take her back to surgery and this time to remove the full skin layer plus adhering fascia and muscle. In total, around thirteen square inches of tissue were removed. This time, the surgery was successful. No more black areas appeared, and the patient went on to full recovery. Similar cases have been reported throughout the years, and surgery is generally the only way to effect a cure, even with improved antifungal therapies.

Another aspect of this organism and other fungal species is when a patient is immunocompromised or immunosuppressed as in organ transplants. A friend of mine had undergone liver transplantation and recovered well. He became a spokesman for transplantation and would give talks based on his experience and encourage people to become organ donors. But after several years, his liver failed again, and he received a second liver. This surgery did not go as well. He was in and out of the hospital until he went in for a terminal stay. I talked to him by phone and learned they had diagnosed him with a fungal disease that had started in a foot and was rapidly discoloring it and moving up the leg. I told him about similar cases and urged him to have the leg amputated sufficiently high above the encroaching growth. But he had had enough. The quality of life after an amputation and the possibility of liver failure made him decide not to have it done, and he died a few days later.

Later, I learned they had diagnosed him as having cryptococcosis and that it was present in his blood. This, too, is an interesting organism. It is commonly found in bird guano, particularly that of pigeons. It has been shown repeatedly that people can inhale the fungal organisms from the air, especially when disturbed guano is present. One such source has been shown to be the tops of window air-conditioning units where pigeons often roost. Could that be the source of my friend's organism? I decided not to pursue this possibility. The infectious control personnel of that hospital should address such problems.

## CHAPTER 14

# The Case for Direct Preparations

EVERYONE IS INTERESTED IN HAVING their problem diagnosed and fixed as soon as possible. To this end some physicians set up laboratories in their offices. In the early years, perhaps they would only run urinalysis, hematocrit, hemoglobin, and blood smears, depending on their confidence level. Others might develop more lab procedures involving simple chemistry tests, direct examination of body secretions, and Gram stains of pus and sputum. In modern times, it is possible to develop more extensive laboratories using analytic machines and kits. But presently, there are generally large commercial labs available with pickup service for their offices or collection sites to which they can send their patients. Some specimens require examinations to be made as soon as possible because a delay may result in the loss of essential information. Let me give you an example.

One day I was sitting in my office when our receptionist came in and presented me with a physician's order for a KOH prep on a patient. Sometime earlier, this laboratory had collected some specimens from patients, although doing so was normally reserved for the physician. I had canceled this practice largely for liability reasons. However, I had been asked personally and had given permission to some physicians to collect certain specimens, such as skin scrapings for fungi, or to obtain throat cultures. I did, however, always refuse to collect "personal" specimens and insisted if the doctors wanted me to examine such they could collect it and have the patient bring it directly to the lab, keeping it warm during transit. This is particularly important for such specimens as vaginal secretions, as the trichomonads in particular would rapidly die when the temperature dropped. Then they could not be differentiated easily from white blood cells. Also, some organisms, such as the gonococcus, also rapidly die off. *Candida* species do not die rapidly and are among the most common causes of vaginosis and what has been commonly called thrush, although this is not a correct term. Thrush can be found in the mouth, in the vagina, and under the breasts, especially when that area is moist. It is not unusual to find it in babies also. Thrush—candidiasis—is a thick, white coating of the tongue and at the corners of the mouth. The organism can be easily identified upon direct examination of the material, and most of the time physicians will order the KOH preparation to show this. But for reasons already stated, I will not use KOH except for hair, skin, and nails. So when the request came for a KOH prep on this patient, I suspected the physician was anticipating that the cause of her ailment was candidiasis.

I agreed to see the patient. She came into my office with her husband and appeared to me to be quite nervous. It turned out that she had a lesion near the tip of her tongue, which she'd had for some time and which was causing her difficulty in speaking. It was about half the size of a dime, very deeply grown, and the surface was a heavy white material. The rim was red. It certainly looked like it might be candidiasis. I got a sterile tongue blade and told her I would like to scrape this lesion, and it might be somewhat painful. She agreed. It was a little difficult to get the material, but I obtained some and went directly to the lab. I washed some off into a drop of saline on a glass slide, placed a cover slip over it, and examined it. I fully expected to find the pseudohyphae characteristic of *Candida* species. I was surprised to put it mildly. No pseudohyphae were present, but there, swimming vigorously around, were trichomonads. Now trichomonads are quite commonly found in vaginal secretions and can be sexually transmitted, but to find them in the tongue was extremely rare. If I had used KOH, the trichomonads would have been immediately killed and appeared as white blood cells. And the treatment for trichomonads and candidiasis are entirely different. The reason the lesion had continued to develop was it was not being properly treated. I immediately called the physician. He, too, was astonished with the result, and he ordered the proper treatment for trichomonads. The patient soon was cured, and the lesion gradually cleared up.

The most common species of trichomonads is *Trichomonas vaginalis*, but there are others too. They all appear essentially the same microscopically, and there are no practical culture methods to isolate them on solid media to conduct further tests, as with bacteria and fungi. There is a method whereby specimens can be placed into a broth medium to isolate them when they are in small numbers. We have used this to isolate a trichomonad but never have found an identification method.

We did not make any effort to determine where the trichomonads had come from, as that is not my field of study. I have never seen another case like this, but it does illustrate the problem. Use of KOH with vaginal specimens could also give the same results (i.e., trichomoniasis would not be diagnosed but would simply appear as an increase of white cells).

Direct examination of vaginal fluids also can identify vaginosis caused by bacteria, which also, incidentally, can be suspected from the presence of a fishy odor. This is caused by small bacteria that cluster around epithelial cells giving them a hairy appearance—clue cells—and actively swimming around. KOH would destroy this, although it does not destroy the yeast cells and pseudohyphae.

Since it is a simple test and readily available in any office that has a microscope, I recommend it, provided the person examining the material is sufficiently well trained to recognize the organisms present. And it does not require oil immersion microscopy, either.

Gram stains are different. These require better microscopes with oil immersion capacity and increased skill in preparing the smears. It is also essential that the person examining the slide has experience and training to recognize what he or she sees.

## CHAPTER 15

# Actinomycetes, Streptomycetes, and Nocardia

THESE ARE VERY INTERESTING ORGANISMS. In some aspects, they are similar, but a major difference is that actinomycetes are anaerobic organisms, but streptomycetes and nocardia are aerobic. Special media and incubation conditions are required to isolated actinomycetes, whereas the others grow handily on media routinely used for the isolation of fungi. These organisms are transitional between bacteria and fungi but in the routine laboratory are normally handled in the mycology section.

Actinomycosis has appeared in literature by the name commonly used for it in cattle: "lumpy jaw." It was once thought that people picked up this condition from cattle indirectly by chewing on a piece of hay that had been in contact (think drooled on) with an infected cow. When I was a boy, we lived on a farm, and when it was haying time, we boys would follow the men around. We observed that the men would frequently walk along the lane, reach down, pull out pieces of timothy hay, and stick them in their mouths. We would emulate them and stick the ends of the stalks into our mouths and push them into the gum line between the teeth. The theory was that a cow infected with lumpy jaw might have deposited some of the organisms onto the stalk of hay, and a person who picked that piece of hay thereby inoculated it into his mouth and might also develop actinomycosis. Humans do become infected with actinomycetes but not by that means.

Many of these stories came before the development of good anaerobic culture methods. With good anaerobic methods, studies of the "normal" flora—*commensal* is the better term—of the mouth proved species of actinomycetes are part of the commensal flora of the mouth. To further demonstrate the association with cattle, the most common species isolated from infections caused by it was named *Actinomyces bovis* (or *israelii*, after the man who described it).

Actinomycetes have been found in abscesses, in mouth lesions, and in the lungs. Quite commonly in the lung lesions, a piece of a tooth, perhaps aspirated during a dental procedure, is found. It might be perplexing to think of the lung as having anaerobic (lacking air) conditions, but it occurs by conditions walling off part of the lung around extraneous material, such as the piece of tooth.

Actinomycetes also has another interesting circumstance: it can grow and penetrate tissue such that it can tunnel out through the lung and into the surrounding tissue. It grows in clumps of thin mycelia much smaller than fungi but has clubbed ends. This feature differentiates it from the nocardia and streptomycetes. The clumps, called sulphur granules, are yellow and range in size from pinpoints to large balls. These can be examined microscopically with the direct prep techniques described earlier. On a Gram stain, they are gram-positive filaments and in this aspect are no different from the nocardia and streptomycetes. But it can be difficult to see these on a Gram stain, as the granules just roll off during the preparation of the slide. If the granules are seen in sputum or fluids drawn from the lungs (thoracentesis or pleural fluid), they should be examined directly and then very carefully teased apart or squashed and gently processed to avoid the washing-off problem.

A young man had developed pulmonary problems resulting in accumulation of fluid in his lungs, which required placing a drain into his left lung. The initial drain plugged up, and a much larger drain was put in. It was successful in draining out the accumulated fluid, but the appearance of the fluid was quite amazing. No one recognized what was happening, as it is a rare condition and had not been observed by any of the staff present.

Some of the fluid arrived in our laboratory, and the material was set up for culture, Gram stain, and direct exam. The latter showed balls of thin mycelia with clubbed ends (i.e., resembling actinomycetes). I was invited to go to the patient's room where I found him in good spirits, as he was feeling better with the pressure being removed along with the accumulated fluid. The tube ran from his chest to a bag hanging from his bed rail. All along the tube sulphur granules suspended in the fluid rolled down into the bag. Subsequent anaerobic cultures (these organisms require from a week to ten days to appear) did grow out *Actinomyces bovis*, but the appropriate antibiotic was started based on the appearance of the granules, the direct prep, and the Gram stain. The patient recovered fully.

A man in his late twenties was referred to the infectious-disease unit of our large teaching hospital with an acute infection of his right elbow. It seemed to be a classic example of an abscess, most probably cause by *S. aureus* or an anaerobic infection, which frequently has mixed etiology. These conditions should be treated by incision and drainage with concurrent intravenous antibiotics given for ten days to three weeks. But this had been done, and the wound had shown minimal improvement—thus, the referral. Our infectious-disease physicians repeated the initial studies but added requests for fungal and acid-fast studies for completeness.

We processed the specimen per protocol, which included doing a Gram stain and an acid-fast stain along with the cultures. The Gram stain showed many white blood cells and long strands of thin septate gram-positive filaments. These could be streptomycetes or nocardia, but they were too thin to be fungal elements. The difference between these two is that streptomycetes are not acid-fast, but nocardia is. We proceeded to perform a Ziehl-Neelsen stain, using a slight modification of the original procedure. The material was spread onto a glass slide and allowed to dry thoroughly. Then it was heated gently to fix the material onto the slide and placed on a staining rack over a pan or the sink. A piece of filter paper cut to fit the slide but *not* large enough to stick over the edge was placed on it, and then the primary stain was flooded onto the slide. A wood stick (we used throat swabs, which were made of wood at the time) was set on fire, held under the slide, and moved back and forth so the stain began to steam. (We didn't want to heat it to boiling.)

The slide was heated for five minutes, which usually required three sticks, one after another. We washed the stain and paper off with a gentle stream of water and then flooded acid-alcohol over the slide until no more red stain came off. (This gives much better results than flooding the slide with acid-alcohol and waiting a specified time before rinsing it off.) The slide was rinsed and then flooded with methylene blue for one minute. This gave a nice blue background on which the red organisms (if they were bacteria like TB, they were called red snappers by some) showed up very clearly. If you don't use the filter paper, the slide may have many background stain particles, which make it more difficult to see the organisms. Nonacid-fast organisms will stain blue. Many laboratories use the auramine-rhodamine fluorescent method as the standard method for acid-fast organisms as we did. It is a good method, but it does require a special microscope, and there are some isoniazid-resistant organisms that do not stain with this method. I found the Ziehl-Neelsen method to be better when checking for nocardia.

In the acid-fast stain of our patient, many red filaments appeared. It was nocardia. It took several days of incubation before the typical rough, raised, orangish colonies began to appear. (One may also notice a distinct odor of dirt, as in a freshly plowed field.) Further studies on the isolate gave us enough information to identify the isolate as *Nocardia asteroides*, the most common pathogen in the genus. There are several more species that don't normally cause disease and another, *Nocardia brasiliensis*, that is pathogenic. But in all cases in which a species of nocardia or streptomycetes is isolated, they must be considered to be the causative agent or perhaps contributory. As soon as we had a positive result on the acid-fast smear, we called the physicians who instituted the appropriate antibiotics, and the patient was cured.

This case was presented in infectious-disease rounds to the visiting infectious-disease physician from another teaching hospital and was one of the few cases we ever knew him to not get as the primary diagnosis. But he knew we wouldn't present him a usual case of abscess just to hear him discuss the recommended treatment regimen, so down at the end of his list of possible pathogens, he made a slight reference to such organisms as nocardia. This, however, was one of the rare instances of *Nocardia asteroides* causing an acute infection. Nocardia would usually produce a more chronic infection as shown in the next case.

The patient had chronic, persistent pneumonia-like symptoms: chronic cough with low-grade fever, malaise, and loss of weight. Routine bacterial cultures did not show any pathogens, but these culture plates are not held for a long time. Repeat specimens were obtained and submitted for fungal and acid-fast studies. No acid-fast rods were found on the smears, but there were some long filaments that were acid-fast. The processing of sputa for mycobacteria will destroy most other organisms, so the cultures were negative.

The fungal cultures did begin to show growth after a week. There was also the slight odor of dirt coming off the cultures. (When I first studied bacteriology, the odor of cultures was included as part of the description of certain organisms. Experienced microbiologists can recognize the odors of such organisms as proteus, pseudomonas, and haemophilus and the dirty-sock smell of staphylococci. They also know enough to not open a plate that has fungal growth on it in the open. It was standard practice to crack open a plate and carefully smell the odor coming off the plate. The odor could give a clue as to what to look for on the plate. But, unfortunately, the government decided, owing to the potential of a technologist becoming infected by smelling the plate, to "outlaw" this practice. Now technologists cannot do this, but sometimes the odor is so strong as to be inescapable. The odor is also sometimes present in a patient, and a knowledgeable physician or nurse will also recognize it. Streptomycetes are found in the soil and are the cause of the classic dirt smell. They are pathogenic to plants (e.g., the cause of "scabs" on potatoes) but were also the source of many early antibiotics. In fact, the world has been searched over for new species of streptomycetes from which the researcher hopes to find the next magic bullet. The oceans were searched, and one such antibiotic came from the sewage effluent going into the Mediterranean Sea. The antibiotic streptomycin was named that as it came from *Streptomyces griseus* and still has special uses.

Since cases of pulmonary nocardiosis are extremely rare and make for interesting discussions, this case was to be presented to the medical grand rounds in the Ether Dome. I was in my animal farm, checking on the many guinea pigs we kept there for testing with clinical species being checked for tuberculosis, when the head pulmonologist entered from the opposite door. He was one of the top pulmonologists in the country. He was looking for me. It was almost time for the grand rounds to start, and he asked me to come with him and hear him discuss the case. I did not want to go, but he persuaded me giving me one of his white lab coats to wear as we did not have time for me to go back to my lab to get my coat.

The Ether Dome was full as usual. There were a couple of chairs in the wings of the stage, and I sat there and listened to the first case. Then the case of the patient with nocardiosis was presented. All the clinical symptoms, the lab test, and the X-rays were shown. Then it was Dr. A.'s turn to discuss the case. I listened fascinated with the discussion and the distinguished audience, including the very famous Dr. Paul Dudley White, who was sitting in the front row. But to my great surprise, Dr. A. turned and pointed to me, saying, "And Mr. Bump is here to discuss the laboratory aspects of this organism. Mr. Bump." And I got up and gave a short lecture describing what we did to isolate and identify nocardia. I was a bit upset, and after the rounds concluded, Dr. A. thanked me and kind of laughed. "Surprised you, didn't I?" I shook my head. "Would you have come if I asked you to do this?" The answer was not without time to prepare, which I didn't have. "You did a good job, thanks."

Later that day, my boss told me he had heard about my performance and congratulated me on it. This case was probably published, but I don't think you would find my name listed, as I did not have a doctorate at the time. It is probably listed as "remarks by a laboratory technologist."

A little later, one of the newer ID physicians came to my lab and asked me what I could tell him about nocardia. I spent some time with him, not only telling him but also showing him both slides and cultures. He had no experience with the organism and only knew about cases he had read about in the literature. Later that week, my boss came and told me to come along with him, as we were going to another unit of our hospital complex for one of its rounds. We sat in the middle of the third or fourth row in an amphitheater. The case was nocardia, and when it was time for a discussion of nocardiosis, the convener introduced the speaker as "our resident expert in nocardiosis." You guessed it. The physician I had spent the time talking to about nocardiosis rose, went to the podium, turned around, and was eyeball to eyeball with me. He sort of blanched but proceeded to give my lecture to the audience.

My boss laughed afterward. "I knew he had gone to see you about this and thought you might like to see how he did." Such situations inspired me to go back to college and earn my doctorate, and after I did, I was called on to speak for myself.

## CHAPTER 16

# *Haemophilus influenza*
# before the vaccine

*HAEMOPHILUS INFLUENZAE* (*H. FLU*) IS an organism with great historic significance as well as personal significance for a great many people. Fortunately,
with the development of a vaccine for the most common pathogenic serotype B (Hib), the incidence of infection and death has been greatly
decreased.

During World War I, there was a pandemic of viral influenza.
What is not as well known is that this epidemic was a double whammy:
Most of those getting influenza at that time also were infected with
*H. flu*. At that time, there were no antibiotics nor was there any real
knowledge of viruses, and therefore, no cure was available. A strain of
the influenza virus (swine flu) has since that time been associated with
large outbreaks, but it is not the scourge that it once was because the
*H. flu* can be eliminated with appropriate antibiotics and most people
are now immunized against it.

Bacterial influenza with associated infections such as otitis media,
sinus infections, meningitis, and at times throat infections was very
common among young children. But it isn't as common among adults,
probably because of the development of antibodies from the exposure to
the organism during childhood. In fact, the dean of infectious-disease
physicians in New England, in his lecture to medical students, would
state that one should not look for *H. influenzae* in throat cultures, and

we did not do so in our laboratory. *H. influenzae* do not grow on blood agar plates unless there are colonies of *Staph. aureus* present, and then they grow in the zone of hemolysis as satellite colonies. To routinely cultivate *H. flu* from a culture, chocolate agar must be used. This was routinely done with such specimens as nasal, sputum, any "sterile" fluids, and bronchial aspirations. (Note: If *H. influenza* was detected in throat cultures because of the satellite phenomenon, that would be reported to the physician. It would be up to him or her to consider this result in the assessment of the patient.)

But there can be exceptions to any rule. One day, a physician requested that we look for *H. flu* in the throat culture of an adult. The technician setting up the cultures noted the request but, since we had the policy of not doing this in throat cultures, did not add the required chocolate agar plate. Nor did the tech notice it was a handwritten request from the dean of infectious diseases and the head of our ID department. The result was reported as commensal flora (i.e., no pathogens including *H. flu* were present).

Dr. W. came storming into the lab after he had been informed by phone that we had not even looked for the *H. flu*. He stormed into my office waving the requisition slip at me and threw in onto my desk. "What the hell is the matter with you people? I ordered a throat culture for *H. flu*, and you didn't do it. What's going on?'

Now I had worked with him for several years. Had gone to his home for journal club. I was aware of his enormous temper but also of his huge intelligence, memory, and willingness to listen to facts. My response was, "An infectious-disease specialist has stated in lectures that *H. influenzae* is not a pathogen in the throats of adults, and I respect his opinion."

He stopped, and a smile crossed his face. He knew I meant him. "Well, yes, he's right, but there may be exceptions. This patient has an extremely red throat, and it is exquisitely painful. I have seen such throats caused by *H. influenzae* in the past. Would you mind looking for it this time?"

"No, sir, we'd be happy to do so. Any time you suspect an exception to the rule we'd be happy to do it. Just be sure to add to the requisition to look for *H. flu*." He recollected the specimen and wrote in please look for *H. influenza*. And we did, and it was present. He treated the patient appropriately, and the cure was soon effected. From that day on, whenever there was a suggestion that an organism might be from an unusual source, the requisition indicated such, and we would adjust our culture regimen to effect the change requested. By working closely together, we could find other unusual pathogens and make significant diagnoses. Some of these did make their way into print, and we were credited for such assistance. This is not always done—that is, a patient practically never learns that an astute technologist had found a causative agent the physician hadn't even suspected so that a diagnosis, treatment, and cure were found. When hiring technologists, I would ask them if their egos were such they required receiving acknowledgment of their work, as it seldom occurs. Although it isn't unusual for the nursing staff to receive—rightfully so—flowers and candy from an appreciative family or their family, the laboratory staff rarely get such recognition. But there have been some cases in which we have been involved that the physician has come to the lab or called and thanked us for our work, and for that we are grateful.

## An Unusual Presentation of *H. influenzae*

One such case occurred when I came to the Owosso (Michigan) Memorial Hospital. One of the long-time pediatricians had an unusual case. A young child had a severe sore throat and congestion. The child could hardly breathe. In fact, she could not breathe lying down and could only draw breath while sitting up. The pediatrician (Dr. B.) ordered a throat X-ray and observed what was called the "thumb sign": the uvula was greatly enlarged and looked as if a thumb was sticking down in the throat, obstructing the trachea. There had been reports of this in the literature, and one of the causative agents was *H. influenzae*. In young children we did include chocolate agar plates, and we knew this could be causing disease in them. The culture was positive for *H. flu*, and Dr. B. continued the therapy of choice, which at the time was ampicillin and chloromycetin. Now chloro is also toxic; it depresses the bone marrow and should not be used in children if possible, and if it is, it should not be for long. Before this toxicity (Gray syndrome) was attributed to the chloromycetin, many children may have been lost to it. It is irreversible. We had a patient admitted to our hospital long after this fact was well known. In fact, the diagnosis of depleted bone marrow was a shock. That it was because of chloromycetin made it even more so. The patient was an itinerant farm worker. He started, as many did, in Florida and followed the work up the coast to New England. He'd had an infection earlier—I don't know the particulars of the first case—and had been treated successfully with chloro. Since it had worked that time, every time he felt ill he would get a scrip for chloro. Actually, he could fake such orders in some way and continue to get the prescription filled. Part of this was because he was an itinerant worker and did not have a family physician. This was fifty years ago; I don't think it would be possible now.

We had developed and used a two-tube system of testing all isolates of *H. flu* for susceptibility to ampicillin and chloromycetin and naturally did so in this case. Ampicillin-resistant *H. flu* was known at the time, and so the chloro was added until we knew that the isolate was susceptible to ampicillin. If it was, then the chloro was discontinued. In this case the isolate was susceptible, the chloro was dropped, and the patient recovered without further incident.

Dr. B. was quite interested in publishing this case, as a search of the literature showed it to be rare, and none of the reports had included the susceptibility testing method we used. The case was written up and submitted for publication. However, it was rejected, as it was only one case. I suspect that part of the reason was that it originated from a small hospital and not a major medical center. But about six months later, the same journal published an article about the same type of patient, but this time there were six cases, and the article came from a major medical center. It was too bad our case couldn't at least have been included in that report. Now it is very common to see "a case of *xyz* (a newly named organism or one rarely if ever reported previously) and search of the literature" being reported. In fact, I have had a couple of those published. The rejection letter said it didn't add to the literature, but the journal was wrong, in that the method of susceptibility testing had not been reported previously, and perhaps the earlier notice might have helped other laboratories.

## CHAPTER 17

# "Cocci" in a Northern Mexican Patient

IT IS NATURAL FOR AMERICANS to shorten or abbreviate names, especially if they are difficult to pronounce, as is true with the fungal disease coccidioidomycoses caused by the fungus *Coccidioides immitis*. It has several other nicknames, such as valley fever and Rift Valley fever. It is endemic in just a few areas of the world that have a specific type of soil. One of these is the southwestern United States, including Arizona, New Mexico, and California. It is also found in northern Mexico and in parts of South America. But is not found in the northeastern United States, and therefore, if a laboratory there isolates this organism, there must be some connection with the endemic area.

The organism lives in the top layers of soil and can be found around prairie dog tunnels. During the wet season, it grows along the surface of the ground, but with the arrival of the dry season, the organism tends to grow down into the soil. And owing to the unusual nature of the organism, which forms alternating arthrospores with a hollow weakened area between them, it can easily break up with friction, air currents, and wind gusts. In this manner, the organism spreads throughout the environment and then can be inhaled by any breathing animal, including humans. It does not take very many endospores to cause pulmonary disease. It can also enter scratches and wounds and produce local lesions. Many people catch a mild form of the disease, which allows them to develop immunity and to recover with minimal damage, believing perhaps that they have gotten the flu.

However, it sometimes goes on to produce much more severe diseases, such as meningitis, and can also result in death. In this way, it is like several of the fungal diseases, and the signs and symptoms are quite similar. One of these is cryptococcosis. "Crypto," however, is found in many parts of the world. It is more usually associated with pigeons and other birds, as the causative agent, *Cryptococcus neoformans*, grows readily in the guano and is transmitted through breathing.

Since these diseases are rare and sometimes can be difficult to diagnose, when such organisms and diagnoses are suspected, it brings a sense of excitement into the clinical field, and there is also a certain sense of competition between physicians and services to successfully diagnose and treat these infections.

One day as I was working in my laboratory, the door burst open, and several men came through the door, one clutching a plastic specimen tube in his hand. One was the head of our laboratory; with him were one of the infectious-disease experts on staff, a couple of residents, and Dr. P., one of the best know neurologists in the area and, for that matter, in the country.

"Dr. P. has a specimen he'd like you to look at for us. It's from a patient he saw on consultation in Mexico. And if there is enough specimen, please culture it."

Dr. P. had a big smile. He had diagnosed his patient with cryptococcosis and started him on amphotericin B—standard treatment at the time. He wanted to show his infectious-disease colleagues a case they probably hadn't seen previously. However, they didn't wait around for me to set up the examination but happily went on their way.

As soon as possible, I centrifuged the specimen, poured off the fluid, and made an "India ink" preparation. This is done by placing a small drop of a special India ink—Pelikan brand—on a slide and a small drop of the concentrate next to it, and then carefully placing a cover slip on it. I always put the edge of the cover slip touching the slide on the ink side and then slowly lower it so the ink flows into the fluid. By this means there is a gradient of too much ink to not enough. If there are organisms there, the ink particles—ink is a suspension of particles and not a solution—will surround it. *Cryptococcus neoformans* in patients is almost always a yeast-like organism that is surrounded by a thick capsule. The ink particles are unable to penetrate the capsule, and therefore, the organism is seen as a round circle of light. The yeast cell is obvious, and the capsule is also obvious. However, there are other structures that form a halo, especially other yeast, white blood cells, and starch particles. Therefore, it isn't that unusual for someone who is not especially experienced to call one of these particles "positive for cryptococcus."

That seemed to be the case here. I did not find cryptococci but did see false-positive structures. I knew this would be a problem. I would be telling all those experts, and Dr. P. too, that the diagnosis was incorrect. Then the questions would be what the real diagnosis was and whether the patient was on a very toxic antifungal agent inappropriately. I made the call and got a flurry of responses from all the physicians involved. My boss came in, and I showed him the specimen. He believed me. But could there be an explanation? One of the possibilities was that the specimen had been a couple of days in transit. With that idea in mind, Dr. P. flew down to Texas, where the patient had been moved (we had been told the man owned half of northern Mexico), did another spinal tap, and immediately flew back to Boston.

I examined the fresh specimen and again did not find cryptococci. I set up fungal cultures, including putting the supernatant fluid into a tube of broth. No growth appeared in the first week, which is what we would expect with cryptococcosis, nor the second week. But during the third week, a couple of fuzzy colonies appeared in the broth tube. I removed these, put them onto solid Sabouraud agar slants, and waited for the growth to develop. It appeared to increase in size in a couple of days but did not take the appearance of a yeast-like growth—raised, rounded, smooth, and creamy appearing—although it was still fuzzy. At this time, I notified all concerned that probably a nonyeast fungus was starting to grow.

Dr. P. called and told me I would get a free trip to Mexico if I could identify the organism. I told him I would do so, but it would take time for the fungi to develop the necessary fruiting structures to identify them. I would do it as soon as possible.

Then I did a bad thing. Slow-growing fungi should not be examined without taking special precautions to prevent the spores from getting into the air and into the lungs of the examiner. One way is to layer the slant with a sterile fluid and then extract a piece of the growth for microscopic examination. Another is to wear a biosafety hood. I did neither, but proceeded to cut out a piece of the agar, including the fungal growth, and to carefully place it into a drop of lactophenol cotton blue and cover-slip it. I placed it under the microscope with moderate magnification. To my absolute astonishment, the typical arthrospores of *Coccidioides immitis* came into view. I had my identification, and Dr. P. had his diagnosis. And the best part of this was that the treatment was the same: amphotericin B.

After the diagnosis, Dr. P. went back to Texas. By means of an Ommaya shunt, he could place the amphotericin B directly into the patient's ventricles, and the man soon responded. A cure was achieved. But, I regret to say, I never got my trip to Mexico.

Serum from the patient was sent to a special laboratory in California for serological testing, and a high titer against coccidioidomyces was found, further confirming the diagnosis.

This case was presented to medical grand rounds and was well received.

## COCCIDIOIDOMYCOSIS IN BOSTON?

This was not the only case of coccidioidomycosis we saw in Boston. The second case, although easily diagnosed by growing the fungus from sputum specimens submitted for culture, could not be explained in a Boston resident. There was no history the patient had ever left the New England area. Where did the organism come from?

Epidemiology is an exciting field, especially when it involves single cases or small outbreaks. The initial phase includes a good history of the patient, including travel, work, food consumed, and contacts with other people. This patient worked at Logan International Airport in Boston which, of course, has airplanes arriving from all parts of the globe. But the patient did not work with travelers directly, and there had been no similar cases reported. Also, this disease is not passed from person to person. Besides, the patient worked in the freight area of the airport. In fact, his job was using a forklift to unload freight off the freight planes, and some of the flights came in from areas where cocci were endemic. We discovered that, as the loads were removed from the plane, it was not unusual for large amounts of dirt and dust to come flying out, and the forklift operators did not wear masks. We did not actually culture the dust from these planes, but we knew that dust carried these spores, and there was no doubt he could have been exposed in this manner.

## CHAPTER 18

# Deli Diarrhea

SALMONELLA "SPECIES"—MORE THAN TWENTY-TWO HUNDRED serotypes—can cause several types of disease, but the one they are probably most commonly associated with is diarrhea. These species are found worldwide and in many different animals and sources in the environment. In 2008 and 2009, there was an outbreak of more than five hundred known cases and several deaths in which the source was found to be peanuts. In an even more recent outbreak, the source was cantaloupe. But the incidence of salmonellosis is far less than it was in the past, owing to higher standards of food processing and monitoring. Also, handwashing and cooking food to temperatures sufficient to kill the organisms have been stressed. The common practice for clinical laboratories after isolating salmonella is to have it typed. In the 1950s and 1960s, most of the larger labs screened an isolate for identification purposes with a polyvalent antiserum A-O and then with the individual groups common at the time. Once identified, the isolate would be submitted to the state health department for serotyping and the health department, in turn, would send it on to CDC for complete evaluation if necessary. In this manner, widespread outbreaks could potentially be identified to a common source, as with the peanuts.

We practiced this in Boston. One hospital at which I worked had isolated an unusual isolate from a patient and forwarded it to the commonwealth's health department. It was identified as a serotype that had been found in enough other patients for them to have begun an investigation.

This investigation finally centered on one of the larger delicatessens in the downtown Boston area (one in which I had eaten in previously).

Once this had been identified as the probable source, the next step was to evaluate the restaurant and the personnel. The store was inspected and found to be in excellent condition (i.e., clean, well-lighted, and with proper refrigeration and cooking). A survey of the personnel, however, revealed that one of the men who prepared sandwiches had chronic diarrhea. The lab obtained stool specimen, which was positive for the same *Salmonella* serotype. The employee was put on sick leave and given treatment to eliminate the organism; he would not be allowed to return to work until he had three subsequent stool cultures with negative results (i.e., no *Salmonella*). The outbreak was stopped.

Several months went by, and we found no more cases of diarrhea with that organism, although we did have other isolates. One day, the technologist working the bench handling stool specimens came to me with a small square of cardboard in hand. On it was a sample of an isolate from a patient showing the same group as we'd seen in the outbreak. We immediately informed the health department and sent the isolate to them. The next day, we heard from them that the isolate was the same serotype as the "deli outbreak" isolate. An inspector went back to the deli, and there was our carrier, hard at work behind the counter. The deli had difficulty finding an experienced sandwich man, and he needed the work and had not reported having diarrhea. However, people can carry the pathogen asymptomatically. The employee had to be let go. The department of health told the restaurant owner not to rehire him unless and until he was cleared by their department.

We did not have a repeat of the outbreak. Either the employee finally was cleared of his carrier state, did not return to the local restaurant business, or went somewhere else with his problem.

## CHAPTER 19

# Shigellosis in Boston

IN ADDITION TO THE NOTORIOUS *Salmonella* species, there are several other genera of gram-negative rods that can cause diarrhea. One of the most common is *Shigella*, named after Japanese microbiologist Shiga. It is commonly transmitted by means of water that is contaminated with feces from infected animals, especially humans. It is of a low-grade infectivity, and the diarrhea comes on rapidly with intense, low abdominal pain, large amounts of gas, and violent explosive diarrhea. It is no fun. I speak from personal experience.

I was invited to give a talk at a conference for representatives of a pharmaceutical house at a New England resort. One of the typical retreats where the reps come to wine and dine and learn more about their products and how to present them to clients. Along with the technical sessions, there is also time to golf, sail, swim, or do whatever the resort might offer.

One of the selling points of any antibiotic is how well it is performing in local hospitals against the isolates they test. And that was why I was there for the day. After presenting my talk, we went off on a power boat for a short trip around the bay on which the resort was located. On that cruise, I had a soft drink cooled with ice. When we came back, it was lunchtime, but it was a quick lunch featuring sandwiches and salad. I chose a BLT. All other meals I had before and after were made with food that was not raw and had been properly cooked.

The following night, I woke with severe abdominal pain and soon had explosive diarrhea. This went on all night, and I used all means at hand to resolve my situation. However, I had to go to work and moderate my labors to accommodate the situation. But as a microbiologist, I knew I could find out the cause of my dilemma by culturing my own stool specimen, which I did. The results: *Shigella flexnerii*, one of the four species and the most common cause of shigellosis in the area. Knowing this, I also knew I would just have to tough it out, and I did. But I wondered where my organism came from. Checking out my food sources from the past week led me to think that it might have been the BLT, as the lettuce or tomatoes may have been contaminated or the water used to wash them was. The ice used in the soft drink might have been made from contaminated water. It was also possible that one of the food handlers or preparers had been a carrier or was currently infected.

Not wanting to accuse anyone, I did call the pharma rep who had invited me to thank her for the opportunity to speak and for the good time that I did have there. In the process of our conversation, I did ask if anyone had gotten ill there. There was a pause and then the confessions that, yes, several people she had talked to had come down with the "crud." Did I have it? An investigation was planned. I never learned if they found the cause, but the suggestion was there was a contaminated water source.

But shigellosis does not usually cause death or long-term problems and does not normally rise to a critical level in public health, as the next story will illustrate.

Our institution not only covered our hospital, outpatient clinics, and some private patients but also was involved with the setup and management of a neighborhood clinic. This was set in a poorer area of the city and covered the needs of a large population, many of whom lived in crowded high-rise apartments. At the time, they were in good shape, but over the years, they gradually turned into a slum. I would go to the clinic periodically and check with the technologists there, evaluate their needs, and see that they were following proper techniques.

There were also several day-care facilities in the same area that had many four- and five-year-old children not yet enrolled in kindergarten. This is still true. The closeness and high activity of these children gives rise to the opportunity for infections with many differing pathogens. And the time I'm referring to was before most of the vaccines now in use were available.

Back in our main laboratory, we were beginning to see a few isolates of *Shigella sonnei*. And as a couple of weeks went by, they greatly increased in numbers. Our techs were interested and began to keep track of them with the demographics available. Almost all the isolates were from children four and five years of age. We informed the department of health about the increase in numbers. They were not interested. After all, it wasn't unusual for infants like this to have a little diarrhea. The number of cases rose to more than fifty patients, and still the public health department wasn't interested. They were worried that there had been several cases of hepatitis in another area of the city. (I think maybe five.)

At the time, I had a young college student working for me on a part-time basis who was planning on going on to become a nurse. She volunteered to study the problem and began to collect the addresses of the patients and to contact their families for further information, looking for the source. She eventually learned that almost all these infants were attending day-care centers. She obtained the names and locations of these centers and contacted them. They, of course, knew they had kids with diarrhea but not the nature. We could tell them about the organism, how it was transmitted, and how to take precautions to eliminate the source. I don't remember the exact number, but I think the final count came to around seventy-five sick children, and we knew other hospitals and clinics also had similar cases. And all of them were from the same general area. We were not invited to visit the day-care centers involved to do epidemiology and evaluate the possible source of the organisms. And we did not learn if there ever was an investigation, but the epidemic did stop, for which all involved were happy.

There were two factors: This was a poor area of town with little or no political power and four- and five-year-old children have no influence and no voice to speak for them. Our personnel cared and acted to eliminate the problem as, I am certain, the personnel in those day-care centers did as well.

## CHAPTER 20

# Lactobacillus, Yogurt, Dental Caries, and Vaginosis

MY JOB WAS TO CONDUCT experiments and studies my boss was interested in but did not have time to perform himself. We did all sorts of things, some leading to important changes and some of which led to dead ends. One day he came to where I was working with several small containers. He had met with an ob-gyn who had been using a new product to treat vaginosis at the request of the sales representative selling this product. It looked like tomato juice and was said to be a culture of a strain of *Lactobacillus acidophilus*, which today is quite commonly known as the organism responsible for making yogurt. Lactobacilli are slender, nonspore-forming gram-positive rods and are naturally found in such areas of the body as the mouth and vagina. They are normally nonpathogenic, although rare cases have been reported in which an isolate of a lactobacillus species may have produced disease.

Historically, lactobacilli have also related to curing thrush, which is a disease caused by the yeast *Candida albicans*. This is thought to be because lactobacilli produce lactic acid, which is toxic to the yeast. But it isn't because of the acidity, as changing the pH of the mouth with inorganic acid solutions, for example, doesn't work. It requires the organic acid. Some people have tried using yogurt to do this, but not all brands of yogurt have viable organisms. Some yogurt is made simply by adding lactic acid to milk to effect the curdling, resulting in yogurt.

In Appalachia, there are people known as "thrush blowers." (This has been mentioned in some of the novels written about this area.) A person who has developed thrush calls for the neighborhood thrush blower, who comes and blows into the mouth of the patient. This, in some cases, cures the patient. This caused some wonder and deserved study. And the results? The successful thrush blower had many cavities and a mouth full of lactobacilli, which, when blown into the patient, served as an inoculum. The inoculum grew in the yeast-infected mouth, producing lactic acid, and this cured the patient. Acidification of the mouth with inorganic acids does not effect the same results and could possibly cause damage.

It is commonly known by practitioners in the field that when a woman develops vaginal candidosis, it is due to a lack of lactobacilli; therefore this product was developed as a treatment. The ob-gyn had been using it in some of his patients with positive results, but he wanted to verify what was in the product. Now the usual lactobacilli found in vaginal cultures can grow quite easily on the sheep blood agar plates we use, but some strains require special media to cultivate it. One such medium was tomato juice agar, which we did not have and had to special order. Once it was in stock, I inoculated the tomato juice agar and blood agar plates with the product. To our surprise, no lactobacilli grew; in its place was a pure culture of *Bacillus* species. Bacilli are gram-positive rods but are generally much larger and thicker than lactobacilli and are spore-producing organisms. They are very commonly found in dust and dirt. Other than the notorious *Bacillus anthracis*, bacilli are not pathogenic and certainly there was no evidence at all that they would be effective against *Candida* and therefore useful in the treatment of candidosis.

We informed the physician of our results and he, in turn, contacted the company making the product. They also confessed bewilderment at our results and sent us fresh samples and a couple of the pure isolates to make certain the media we were using would sustain the growth. The pure cultures did grow as expected, but the fresh containers were shown to be a mixture of organisms: the lactobacilli and some bacilli.

Our conclusion was that the product had become contaminated with bacilli during the manufacturing process. Since bacilli are spore formers, the spores would develop in the natural sequence of events, but the lactobacilli would gradually die off. We supplied all this information to the manufacturer, who informed us the company was taking measures to correct the problem, but we did not hear back from them. I do not think that this product is in use today. It makes just as much sense to use a douche of natural yogurt to "cure" a case of vaginosis, although this is esthetically not as pretty.

Disease often results when the usual balance of a biological niche is thrown into disarray by external influences. Some organisms can be present in the body and not produce disease unless thrown out of balance; then they do. Yeast falls into this category. It is quite common to find a few yeast colonies in cultures such as the mouth, throat, stool, or vagina without disease.

Lactobacilli are thought to be a major player in the emergence of dental caries. The acids formed—while good at keeping the yeast in check—can attack the enamel of the teeth and allow the caries to begin. There are many different organisms in a so-called "normal" throat, and the balance helps keep the throat free from disease. Actually, we examine throat cultures for the presence or absence of commensal flora and specifically look for the notorious group A streptococcus (*Streptococcus pyogenes*). Other possible pathogens, such as *Staphylococcus aureus*, *Neisseria meningitidis*, *Streptococcus pneumoniae*, and *Haemophilus influenzae*, for example, are not reported unless the commensal flora is greatly reduced or absent and the other pathogen is there in significant numbers. Two exceptions would be if the physician had specifically requested a search for these other pathogens and in young children, in whom *H. influenzae* is significant. Another exception would be the finding of *Neisseria gonorrhoeae* (GC), which can cause pharyngitis and would be reported.

## CHAPTER 21

# *Listeria monocytogenes* and Mrs. Perkins

ONE OF THE MORE INTERESTING but rarely encountered organisms, in my estimation, is that small, slender, nonspore-forming gram-positive rod named after the great microbiologist Josef Lister: *Listeria monocytogenes*. It can be found in strange places, such as coleslaw and other food products from which it colonizes in humans. It has been associated with the condition known as infectious mononucleosis (the kissing disease) but now is known as not causing it. This came about as the inoculation of the organism into the eyes of rabbits resulted in the appearance of large numbers of monocytes, which led to the naming of the organism. It has also been known to cause spontaneous abortions in humans, as it has a predilection for growing in the vagina, owing to certain amino acids present there. And it has been isolated from the elderly with meningitis, especially men. In fact, if we were sent a specimen of cerebral-spinal fluid from an elderly man and found large numbers of white blood cells, we would expect to find small, thin gram-positive rods. A culture would show small beta-hemolytic white colonies. We would also examine the growth by means of a hanging drop preparation for motility, as *Listeria monocytogenes* has a unique motility: end-over-end tumbling. The examination of the organism by special flagellar stains shows a single flagellum at one end of the rod. A Gram stain of any growth from CSF is always made, and this would enable one to differentiate the rods from the round coccoid forms of streptococci that have similar-appearing colonies.

If you grow listeria on nonblood-containing tryptone agar, another phenomenon can be observed in oblique lighting. Listeria appear as ground-glass, bluish-green colonies, while similar colonies of streptococci species are smooth, yellowish colonies. We were interested in demonstrating the presence of listeria in throat cultures and used this technique. Throat cultures that were submitted to our laboratory were also cultured on the tryptone agar and examined by oblique lighting and we did find some. They are very rare and not worth looking for on a routine basis, but one can establish listeria as part of the commensal flora. This can also be done with vaginal cultures.

Working in a hospital in the town in which you live can sometimes present you with highly confidential situations. You can imagine running tests or cultures for sexually transmitted diseases and finding out the patient is someone you know. Confidentiality is paramount, and breaking this is an offense for which employment can and will be terminated. But it also can bring back good memories of times long past.

Findings of rarely isolated organisms cause a stir in the laboratory, and these cultures are shown around, especially to younger technologists and physicians who may never have seen such isolates. For example, tularemia, plague bacillus, brucellosis, pertussis, and listeria would all fit into this category. Isolating some of these organisms requires special methods, and we would not even look for them unless we were told this would be a possibility. In addition, some such isolates would require to immediately notify the attending physician and the infection-control personnel, as it could require immediate institution of specified isolation procedures.

One day, an excited technologist brought a culture plate to me and stated she thought it might be listeria. The isolate was from the spinal fluid of a seventy-plus-year-old lady (which, as I have stated, would be rarer than from an elderly man). We set up the necessary tests, informed the physician, and asked about the case, as it is always interesting to learn about the patient if it doesn't break confidentiality. The patient lived alone in an apartment building in the town in which I had been born and raised. We learned that her neighbor had come by and noticed her apartment door was open. She knocked, heard no reply, and entered. The lady was lying on the floor in her living room, unconscious. She was brought to our hospital by ambulance and emergency-room physicians suspected meningitis. She was immediately tested and started on antibiotics, and everything necessary to treat the meningitis was done. We did a Gram stain on the specimen, and gram-positive rods were reported, so the treatment was appropriate and Mrs. Perkins recovered.

When I looked the case up, I was surprised and saddened to learn that she was our neighbor in my hometown. She had been one of the first to visit our house to see me the day after I was born. Our families had been friends for many years. It saddened me to learn where she had been living, as I had thought she had already passed on. I was able to visit her in her room and we spoke of the times in which we lived, and I learned her impression of life in our town and neighborhood. Her daughter was also by her mother's side and it made it a special visit.

Confidentiality is extremely important in our business and must not be compromised. More than once I have been privileged with information on well-known people and had to plead to having no knowledge to maintain confidentiality. This is a trust to be held in the medical field and must not be broken.

This reminded me of another case in which I was involved.

I had taken a three-week vacation to visit the Baptist Hospital laboratory in Barranquilla, Colombia, both to evaluate and assist in any way I could and to learn from them. I was especially interested in gaining experience in reading blood smears for malaria. Malaria was seen quite regularly there at the time, and that is still probably true. Colombia had a program in which medical personnel went into villages and obtained blood smears from anyone who had a recent history of fever, even if it might not be suggestive of malaria. In this manner, they did discover early emerging cases and could give the patient appropriate medication. There were always many slides to review, and they were not infrequently positive for more than one type of malaria. I could get experience reviewing slides.

Back in Michigan, it was unusual to even get smears to read specifically for malaria and even rarer to find a positive smear. Since I had the added training, any time a hematology technologist found a suspicious smear, he or she brought it to me for confirmation. One day we found a positive smear. We learned that the patient was a woman who had recently been on a safari to East Africa with her husband. She had typical symptoms of malaria and with the positive smear was treated and recovered. Her husband did not have malaria.

That summer I attended my high-school reunion in Flushing, Michigan, where all the classes that had graduated more than twenty-five years before met together. Each class sat together around tables and enjoyed discussing what had happened since their last time together. One of the stories was from a classmate who mentioned going on the safari and "catching" malaria. I asked her about taking the prophylactic medicine recommended for travelers to certain regions, and she admitted that she had missed a dose. That is enough to allow the malarial parasite to get in. I told her I knew of her diagnosis as I had read the smear showing the organism but would have said nothing otherwise.

## CHAPTER 22

# Pseudoepidemics

CONTAMINATION OF MEDICAL MATERIALS, DEVICES, and medications of any type is a very serious problem. Some of these are picked up as an epidemic (e.g., a seeming outbreak of blood infections [bacteremia] with the same organism). These can often be solved in a very short time if the organism is one that is not usually a pathogen to humans but is a common contaminate, such as the *Bacillus* species.

But it is much more difficult if the organism is capable of producing disease, especially in a person who is immunocompromised, or otherwise in a weakened condition. Such organisms are the ubiquitous *Staphylococcus epidermidis* (coagulase-negative staphylococci) and alpha-hemolytic streptococci. This would be easier to resolve if the generally recommended practice of obtaining at least three blood cultures fifteen minutes apart if there is a suspicion of bacteremia or septicemia were followed. However, it is not unusual for a physician to only order one blood culture. Part of this is because of a false sense of economy. One culture is, of course, cheaper than three, but if it leads to a false result and a patient is put onto long-term antibiotic therapy, it can be much more expensive than the three cultures. Coagulase-negative staphylococci are common inhabitants of the skin of humans and, therefore, easily picked up when obtaining a blood culture if the skin has not been properly disinfected. One positive culture out of one must be investigated. But if it is only one culture out of three, it is less likely to be a causative agent or a true bacteremia. Following the recommended procedure, it would be more likely that two bottles were taken for each blood culture. So one bottle out of six would probably be a contaminant, and the physician would also be able to determine from the patient's clinical picture if the one positive bottle was a false result.

But there is the aspect of finding what is normally a true pathogen in only one bottle. For example, if you obtained one blood culture, and the organism that grew out was a serotype of the genus *Salmonella*, that could not be ignored. It would have to be treated until it was determined to be the result of contamination by some very unusual source; it just doesn't happen. It also goes back to the principle mentioned earlier: if you hear hoofbeats, think horses not zebras. One must always keep in mind that there may be a circus in town, and a zebra could have gotten loose. Let me illustrate this with a case.

A young lady was admitted to our hospital in a rural county in Michigan with a fever of unknown origin. A full workup was ordered for her, including three sets of blood cultures. The cultures were positive for gram-negative rods, which would indicate a reason to initiate chemotherapy, and this did happen. We next set up cultures to isolate and identify the organism. After the first twenty-four hours, we found that the organism was a lactose nonfermenter, a group of organisms including *Salmonella*, *Shigella*, and pseudomonads. We set up the usual set of tubed media. (This procedure is no longer done, as it is possible to set up panels to identify gram-negative rods overnight.) The next day, we were totally surprised to find a picture indicating a very rare organism for this part of the country especially: *Salmonella typhi*, the causative agent of typhoid fever. We then went immediately to the serotyping of the organism as *S. typhi* has a distinctive antigen known as the VI factor or virulence. And it was positive. But where on earth could this patient have contracted typhoid fever? We called the physician and learned he thought she had contracted some venereal disease or perhaps had had an ectopic pregnancy, as she had gone to visit her boyfriend and came back ill. He hadn't examined her too thoroughly, or he probably would have noticed the distinct rose spots of this disease that were present.

We were interested in finding out more about this patient. She was too ill to be questioned at the time, but her mother was also anxious to get to the bottom of the story and was willing to provide some of the information. It turned out that the boyfriend and a group of other students from one of our large universities had traveled to a Central American country for an educational program working with the locals. All those students had received the necessary shots for travel in that part of the world, which included typhoid fever. The patient was not part of the group. She had only decided to go there later and had not gotten the recommended shots.

But this did not fully explain the situation. The city and country they were in did not have typhoid fever. We needed more information. The mother found it for us. It seems the group had taken a few days and gone to a neighboring country that had an outbreak of typhoid fever during the time they were there. Our patient hadn't arrived at that time but came later. None of the students who had gotten the vaccine developed typhoid fever, but they could have been contaminated with the organism. Our patient did have close personal relations with her boyfriend. She had probably gotten the organism from him and, lacking the antibody to it, had acquired the infection.

So the conclusion was that she had indeed acquired typhoid fever by contact with her boyfriend and had come home with it. Even one bottle positive for *S. typhi* is significant.

Unusual cases do occur with sometimes obvious causes. Growing a fungus in a blood-culture bottle is unusual. Normally, one does not get a fungemia caused by a filamentous fungus. Yeast, yes, but not filamentous fungi, so if there is a filamentous fungus growing in a blood culture, it is probably a contaminant, and the source needs to be found. Once we received a full IV bottle and tubing along with a set of blood cultures. The patient had been running fevers, and the doctor had not yet identified a source. To our astonishment, we found the IV line from the bottle to be plugged with filaments of fungi. We examined the bottle and found a crack in a rough area of the glass, which made it virtually invisible. The bottle itself was full of fungal filaments, making it look like it was filled with a spider's web. A careful examination of the bottle when it was hung would have shown this. The only time I ever saw fungi in a bottle was when the bottle was cracked. Of course, since almost all IV solutions are now given in plastic bags, this source is no longer found. That does not mean that the solution itself couldn't be contaminated from another source but at least not because of a broken bottle.

We learned that many of the babies in the newborn nursery had shown cultures positive for *Pseudomonas aeruginosa*, which is a water-borne organism of low pathogenicity. It is not unusual to find it causing bladder or urinary-tract infections and pneumonia in older patients. However, these babies were showing positive sputum and throat cultures, and a couple of them developed septicemia. None of them were at-risk babies, but the organism had to be getting to them somehow. The pediatricians were reluctant to start them on antibiotics, as pseudomonads are frequently quite resistant to many antibiotics and would require antibiotics that weren't recommended for use on babies. We had to determine if these were true results or some sort of contamination and, if so, where it originated.

An inspection of the nursery was in order. The first thing I noticed was that the nursery was overcrowded with bassinets. To reach a baby on the far side of the nursery, one would have to push and pull the bassinets around. It was difficult to move around and through them to attend the babies. An inspector from an accrediting agency would certainly have written them up for this violation. The personnel there knew this and were embarrassed by the conditions, but there was little that could be done because of the large number of babies being born there at the time. (The idea of sending a pregnant woman to another local hospital and losing the income was unthinkable.)

I next observed that there were a couple of small water baths in the nursery. Upon questioning, I learned they were used to warm the bottles of milk or formula before giving them to the babies. I watched as an attendant came and retrieved a bottle from the water bath, inverted it, and tested the milk against the inside of her forearm to determine if it was warmed sufficiently but not too much. A very natural thing. But she did nothing to prevent the water clinging to the bottle from running down the nipple and comingling with the milk. I looked into the water bath and could see that the water was very cloudy and could smell the odor of pseudomonads emanating from it. That is not a bad thing if you like a grape-like odor. Pseudomonads generally give off a distinctive sweetish odor. (There are several organisms that can be distinguished by a distinctive odor. Haemophilus is like mouse fur to me; proteus is quite distinct, but I couldn't tell you what to compare it to. You'd just have to learn it. A nursing student once spent some time in my laboratory, and I pointed out these odors and commented that they would also be present in a patient infected with the organism. Years later, as she was making rounds with the infectious-disease physician in a regional hospital, she commented to him as they passed a room that the patient in there must have an infection caused by pseudomonads. He stopped in his tracks. She was correct, of course, but then he knew she had spent time in the lab and put it together. He also used odors to help identify infections.) I obtained samples of the water from the baths and cultured them. They had very high levels of mixed pseudomonads. The nursery staff was instructed to completely dry the bottles before inverting them to prevent the water from contacting the babies, and the epidemic ended. Of course, the water baths were emptied, cleaned, and refilled with fresh water to which disinfectants were added, and they were cleaned thereafter on a scheduled basis. Use of heaters which don't use standing water was also recommended. This should also be a reminder to mothers at home. Don't keep using the same water over and over unless it is brought to a boil to kill off any organisms present. Better still, use it to warm the bottle, then discard it and get fresh water the next time.

# A PSEUDOEPIDEMIC ORIGINATING IN THE MICROBIOLOGY LABORATORY.

This pseudoepidemic ended in what could be described as a miracle but started as a rash of positive blood-culture bottles from random patients. These bottles were positive for *Pseudomonas* species. We began an investigation, as the initial observation showed the patients from whom the specimens had been obtained did not have signs or symptoms consistent with a bacteremia. In most cases, it was only a single bottle and that following our final culture check of previously negative readings.

The lots of the blood-culture bottles were checked and uninoculated bottles run, but none were positive. All bottles were in dated, and there was no correlation of techs, wards, or any other reasonable source.

I began a review of our procedure and found that the bottle tops were always wiped with gauze squares, which were kept in jars of 70 percent ethanol. At the time of the subculture of the bottles, a square was removed, used to wipe off the bottle before the needle was inserted to obtain the specimen, and then discarded. Was it possible that the pseudomonads were in that jar? The alcohol should have killed off the organisms. I sampled the jar and found pseudomonads like those from the positive blood-culture bottles in the alcohol.

Since 70 percent alcohol will burn, I took a small sample and, with a burning swab, attempted—several times—to burn the alcohol, but it always put out the flame. Next, I took the jar to the chemistry department and asked them to tell me the percentage of alcohol that was present; perhaps it had been diluted or mixed incorrectly. The chemist's results were negative (i.e., no alcohol was detected).

We discarded that container, requisitioned a new one, and carefully restocked the gauze squares with 70 percent alcohol. The positive cultures stopped.

We had no definite answer. The biblical turning of water into wine seemed to have been reversed. There was some speculation that an employee—knowing we had been using ethanol—may have done the old trick of taking out the alcohol and replacing it with water so no one would notice the level had gone down. We changed from ethanol to isopropyl alcohol and labeled it as such, and our problem also was gone.

## CHAPTER 23

# Group B Streptococci when it was an emerging pathogen

Steve knocked lightly on my office door, then came in, and sat in the chair in front of my desk. He was a tall, thin young man with wild, long black hair and rugged handsome looks. He hadn't been working for us for very long but did good work and was interested in learning as much as he could to advance his career. Beginning technologists are usually started in one of the less-complicated sections of the workbench and progress through the other benches one by one until they become experienced in all fields of the clinical laboratory. Ours was a major teaching hospital, and the microbiology laboratory was separate from the chemistry and hematology departments. We would usually start a beginning tech in the blood-culture area, although this is one of the most important areas, because it was usually simpler to handle than some other areas. At that time, culture bottles were examined visually at least twice a day, and if there were any suggestion that they were positive—color change, turbidity, gas bubbles present, or floating colonies—the tech would remove a sample, perform a Gram stain, and set up a culture based on the results. In any case, a blood agar plate and a chocolate agar plate would be inoculated. If organisms appeared on the Gram stain, we would call the physician of record with the results. After growth appeared with overnight incubation isolation, the tech performed identification and susceptibility testing. These techniques would be applicable to all other areas or benches of the lab.

Steve had worked his way through the benches and was now working with the genital culture area, which included cultures for gonorrhea. At that time the vaginal cultures were examined for GC, candidiasis, and any predominant organism if present in large numbers. We did not do anaerobic cultures. Gradually, over the years, we added other organisms to the list of potential pathogens, but we adhered to the policy of reporting what was present in the culture without regard to the significance of the specific organism. The significance was left up to the discretion of the physician. But we had noticed an increase in the number of cultures with the presence of group B streptococci.

Now I may need to explain about hemolysis and streptococci. Hemolysis is the dissolving of the red blood cells present in the culture media. It also depends to a certain degree on the kind of blood being used. We used sheep blood, not human blood or horse blood. In sheep blood, there are two kinds of hemolysis: alpha and beta. A third designation, gamma, is also used but gamma is the description when no hemolysis appears, and the blood remains unchanged. Alpha hemolysis is when the red blood cells (RBCs) are partially degenerated, and there is a slight change in the hemoglobin, resulting in a green coloration under and around the colonies. Beta hemolysis is the description when the RBCs are completely dissolved, and there are no RBCs left in the immediate area surrounding the colonies. The most famous streptococcus is the notorious group A beta-hemolytic strep. The grouping of streptococci was developed by Dr. Rebecca Lancefield and is known as the Lancefield groups. Group A strep are the causative agents of strep throat and other, more serious, sequalae to the growth of these strep in humans. But group B has not been as important. The other groups did not match the level of group A either, but some group C and group D strep are quite important pathogens. Group D is also subdivided into enterococci and nonenterococcal group D and are quite common in urinary-tract infections.

What is not as well known is that not all group B streptococci are beta hemolytic. They have a unique colony formation on blood agar plates, appearing as flat, round, white colonies much larger than group A. The color is more of a bluish-white (think skimmed milk) and distinctive to the trained, experienced eye. We had gotten into the practice of checking all those nonhemolytic colonies that gave the appearance of group B strep to make certain and reporting them if they were present in significant numbers in vaginal or cervical cultures. It was regarding these isolates that Steve approached me with a suggestion and a proposal.

How would it be if we could check out the presence of group B streptococci in the "normal" patient as well as those submitted for undisclosed problems? This would require a couple of things. First, it would be an added expense. Could we spend the money? Second, how would we get the normal patient cultures? And third, who would do the work and keep track of the results? It would be my job to take care of all three, but he would also volunteer to do the analysis of results and convince the other techs to continue this work when he wasn't at that bench. I decided to do a literature search and to learn how much of this was known at the time.

I contacted the physician in charge of our well-patient clinic. Clients of this clinic included personnel, medical students who used our clinic, and women coming in for prenatal visits. She was most accommodating, provided we would keep her informed about the results.*

There were quite a few papers published about the indication that group B strep could be pathogenic both to regular patients and to newborn babies but virtually none about the normal carriage of this organism. So we began our study. In a short time, it became evident that a significant number of women were carrying group B streptococci without any evidence of disease. We were also comparing the number of group B strep being found in patients causing some level of infection. A few newborn babies were also being infected. Some of these babies showed evidence of clinical infection almost immediately after birth, but some of them did not develop it until later.

---

* Earlier, we had cooperated with one of the infectious-disease physicians and Dr. R. in the clinic to study pharyngeal carriage of gram-negative rods. This study was published and was one of the first papers to establish the fact that gram-negative rods can be part of the commensal oral flora.

Our results indicated that almost 40 percent of assumed "normal" females were carriers of group B strep. Many papers have been published subsequently, and the reported range of group B carriage is quite wide, but the findings resulted in a change in the way ob-gyns treat these patients. There is a great reluctance to treat a woman who is carrying group B strep with antibiotics while the baby is still in utero because of the potential of harming the baby in some way. However, waiting until the baby shows signs of disease is also not recommended. Now it isn't unusual to begin specific therapy on the mother as she goes into labor so that the organism does not get a chance to gain entry. Treating babies born to group B moms is up to the pediatrician.

In the laboratory, it should now be the policy to look for and report the presence of group B streptococci whether the organism is beta hemolytic or nonhemolytic. We instituted this policy in consultation with our infectious-disease physicians as soon as we had completed this study and saw the high level of group B strep. Steve had done a good thing, and even though we did not get this published, the information was used by our hospital to bring about change. It was also included in Dr. W.'s lectures on streptococci to the medical staff and students.

## CHAPTER 24

# Giardiasis in Shiawassee County, Michigan

*GIARDIA LAMBLIA* IS A SINGLE-CELL protozoan that causes bloating, gas, and diarrhea in humans. It is usually associated with beaver, muskrat, and other such animals that live in or near fresh water in the colder climates of North America. It can be present in the fresh mountain streams downstream from beaver ponds, for example. It is a very distinctive parasite and easily recognized by the trained, experienced technologist. But it is on the rare side of intestinal parasites except in the endemic areas. Shiawassee county is in central Michigan, and beaver haven't been around for many years, but muskrats are quite common. In fact, it was at one time a primary area for obtaining pelts for making fur coats and other items of clothing before these were targets for animal lovers. Other fur-bearing animals, such as mink and raccoon, were also abundant. During the Great Depression, families found muskrat a good source of food. (They also ate woodchuck, opossum, and deer with regularity.) The cases I am about to describe occurred approximately thirty years ago. Perhaps there will be more now, as recently there have been reports of beaver again being found in the county.

When a patient develops diarrhea, the best course of treatment often is to treat the symptoms and give it time. Treatment with antibiotics is not always recommended, as it could result in selecting out resistant types of the organisms, which, if the patient develops systemic disease, would then be much more difficult to treat. But if the diarrhea persists, efforts must be made to determine the causative agent. The standard is to obtain cultures and examine for ova and parasites on three sequential events of diarrhea.

Examining stool specimens for ova and parasites is not among the more enjoyable jobs done in the clinical microbiology laboratory, as you may well imagine. But once the specimen has been processed—which includes washing and centrifuging the specimen to concentrate any parasites—the actual microscopic examination is neither difficult nor usually smelly. It can be boring, though, as they are generally negative in this area of the country. We required the techs to examine both an unstained cover slip and one stained with iodine and to spend fifteen minutes on each slide. When they found something they suspected of being a parasite, most techs would ask for a second tech to confirm or deny the finding.

One day I was called to check out a result and was happy to confirm the cross-eyed appearance of the classic *Giardia lamblia*. Perhaps you wonder about the "happy," but it was because, when we find something interesting like this, it did brighten up the boring aspect of that work bench. Also, finding this meant a diagnosis had been found, and a treatment would be instituted to cure the patient. But in addition, it meant an investigation of the patient's surroundings was needed to find the source and to take measures to eliminate the organism from that source.

The problem continued, in fact, four more times. There were the father, the mother, and three children, and naturally the physician had ordered ova and parasites tests (O&P) three times, so over the next two days, we had a total of fifteen positive specimens. We informed the physician of the results and initiated correct therapy immediately, along with checking into the possible source of the infestation.

This was about half the battle. It seemed there were another five people involved, so we got more and more specimens from the same family as two sisters lived next door to each other and took turns taking care of their children, all with diarrhea. They lived out in the country in a relatively isolated part of the county near one of the small rivers that drained extensive swampy areas. These waters did abound with muskrats. At first, we thought they might have acquired the parasites from playing in or near the stream. It is difficult to demonstrate giardia in such streams as they will be in low numbers, and it would take large amounts of specimen to concentrate to find them. An examination by a county sanitarian found the family had a well for their water source, but the well was located within the one-hundred-year flood plain, as was the home. The construction of the well was such that the spring flooding from melting snow and heavy rains washed into the well and had probably carried with it sufficient contaminated water to contaminate the well. The well was treated, and in the meantime, the families were instructed not to drink any of the water without first boiling it to kill off any parasites and other organisms that might be present.

## CHAPTER 25

# Circumcision

THIS IS NOT A DISCUSSION about the merits of doing circumcisions (circs) but rather a recounting of an outbreak and how to identify the source and correct it. It was a rather easy one to do but very illustrative of a problem that I have encountered several times over my career. The reaction is always the same when a possible outbreak has been identified, especially in post-surgical specimens: it is the environment. And the surgeons especially want the environment to be checked out immediately, but it is almost never the environment, although there are times a pathogen can be found there. The second source they want to check out is the attending staff: nurses, aides, orderlies, and all others who might be passing through the vicinity. All, that is, except the surgeons.

This does not mean that there are not problems associated with the environment, some of which I have already covered, but it is not the pre-dominant source. We routinely cultured areas of the hospital including the kitchen, the OR, the patient rooms, the nursing stations, and the work-rooms. A casual observance of the ER and postsurgical recovery room could show areas of concern. One such would be the curtains dividing the spaces. Look at the end of the curtain about waist high and see if there is a discoloration showing the curtain had not been changed. If you take a culture from that area, it would not be surprising to find organisms includ-ing staphylococci.

We checked drains in the cystoscopy suite and found pseudomonads. We recommended the drains be disinfected, although it is doubtful the organisms caused an infection in the patient above; rather, the urine and so on coming from them was likely nourishing the organisms.

Once the position of infection-control coordinator (or nurse) was established, part of our normal procedure was to furnish them a list of all the patients from whom we isolated a probable pathogen and the antibiogram from all such isolates. The ICC would then go to the ward where the patient was located and determine if the case was a true infection or colonization and if it was nosocomial or community acquired. This would form the basis of the ICC's monthly report to the infection-control committee. It was also sometimes a point of contention with the staff, particularly when the infection rate for each physician and surgeon was made known. Some of this information was difficult to acquire, as there were infections occurring some days after the patient had been released, and unless that patient came back to the ER, we would not know about it. Some hospitals send post cards to the medical staff requesting follow-up on patients, particularly surgeries, but the staff does not return them. It is for that reason I report a small outbreak of infected circumcisions and the follow-up.

It is the normal procedure to circumcise most of the male babies born in the hospital. Sometimes it is done by a rabbi as a ritual circumcision, but it was not in this case. We had an outbreak of *S. aureus* in several of our babies, and the later phage typing showed it to be the same type. An antibiogram of the staph is usually insufficient to determine if they are the same organism. Armed with a list of the positive cultures, it did not take us too long to find that almost all the circs had been done by the same physician. Two other things were observed. Although most of the nurses attending the circs were the same, not one had attended all of them. The physician was observed performing a circ wearing a mask, but it did not cover his nose—just his mouth and chin—and he did not wear sterile latex gloves.

The first thing we did was to obtain nose and hand cultures of all the nurses working on the circumcisions, and they all turned out to be negative (i.e., no staphylococci). Then, even though we knew almost all the infected circs had been done by the one physician, we presented the problem to all the physicians who had performed circs, along with the information that the staff had tested negative, and requested cooperation from them in culturing their noses and hands. They did, and the suspected physician did have staph in his nose and on one of his hands. Once the information was presented under confidential conditions, as was the final report, he cooperated, started wearing gloves, wore his mask properly, and was treated to eliminate the carriage state. The outbreak came to an end, and the whole problem was successfully resolved. It has not always been that easy.

## A Similar Problem but with General Surgical Procedures

At another time in another hospital, we had a problem within the orthopedic unit. It was a large facility with many visiting physicians as well as the resident staff. We went through the usual: it's the environment. Checked and found clean. It's the staff. Checked and no carriers. Now it was time for the physicians and, to no one's surprise, little cooperation. It was easier to get the med students, interns, and residents, as there was a hold over them. When we had 100 percent of them tested and found negative, we persisted in pursuing the senior and visiting staff. We went to the department of surgery staff meeting and presented our information: everyone and everything had been tested except some of them. Most of them lined up for nasal cultures, and all we tested were negative. It came down to two surgeons, one of whom had worked on most of the positive cases. Back to the department meeting and the report that we had tested all but two of them and not found the carrier. The pressure was on and did result in what we needed. One brought in cultures he said came from his nose and hands, but of course, we only had his word for it. He was negative. And finally, the last surgeon was found alone in the doctors' lounge and reluctantly agreed to the cultures and, you guessed it, he was a staph carrier. Presented with the culture evidence, he underwent proper therapy for eliminating the organism. The first check found a few left, and a second treatment regimen was completed successfully. We could go back to the department meeting and declare the source eliminated, and the outbreak came to an end, too.

Another time, we identified a surgeon who had become a carrier and did pass his organism on despite being extremely careful when working on his patients. He was treated several times, but the treatments were never able to eliminate his staph. He decided to give up the surgery part of his practice and, in fact, went on to a teaching position. No one who has devoted his or her life to the practice of medicine would like it to come to an end like this.

## CHAPTER 26

# Conclusions

MANY CHANGES HAVE OCCURRED OVER the forty-plus years I have studied and worked in the field of clinical microbiology. Some of these changes are the result of advances in areas of molecular biology that were practically applied to the clinical field specially to make the identification and susceptibility testing of microorganisms possible. What formerly took many separate tubes of culture media, days of incubation, and additional testing—that is, the identification and susceptibility testing of many organisms—can now be accomplished overnight. Serological identification of causative agents has been simplified, making possible identification of diseases previously unknown. There has also been a great reduction in the number of patients acquiring the diseases that were the most common before the explosion of science following World War II. These include diphtheria, whooping cough, bacterial pneumonia, measles, polio, and childhood infection caused by *H. influenza* because of the development of vaccines. Smallpox has been eradicated. New pathogens have been discovered and added to the list of clinical diseases. What was common has now become rare, and the organisms previously rarely seen can now be seen on a regular basis. Who knows what the future holds? But what is certain is that the microbes haven't given up. Due primarily to the overuse or inappropriate use of antibiotics, resistant strains of common bacteria can now be deadly, and the development of new antimicrobials is a long, difficult, and expensive process. Yet this must be done so infectious diseases may be overcome.